BALANCE FOR
Busy Moms
Cook Your Way to **Health**

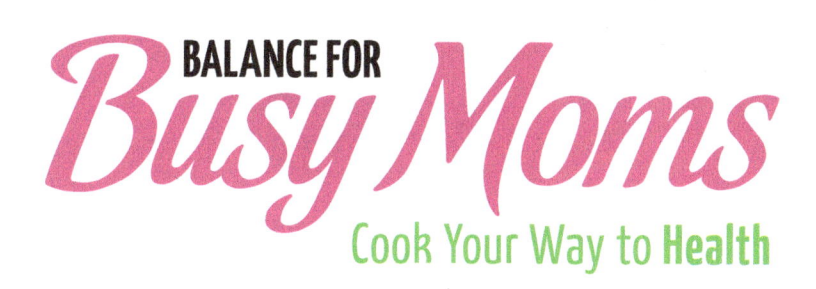

COMPILED BY
HEATHER EDEN

Balance for Busy Moms

Copyright © 2014, Heather Love Eden

All rights reserved worldwide.

No part of this book may be used or reproduced in any manner without written permission. This publication is protected under the US Copyright Act of 1976 and all other applicable international, federal, state and local laws, and all rights are reserved, including resale rights.

CM Publisher
c/o Marketing for Coach, Ltd
Second Floor
6th London Street
W2 1HR London (UK)

www.cm-publisher.com
info@cm-publisher.com

ISBN: 978-0-9928173-5-0

Published in UK, Europe, US and Canada

Book Cover and Inside Layout: Alvaro Beleza

Table of Contents

Gratitude 9

Introduction 11

PRACTICE 1 **The Power of Choice**
By Heather Eden 16

PRACTICE 2 **Listening to Our Internal Cues**
By Jennifer Perry, RNFA, CHHC, AADP 24

PRACTICE 3 **Trust Yourself**
By Lisa Bakosi, MS, CHC, AADP 32

PRACTICE 4 **Lose the Labels, Lose the Weight**
By Sarah Mobry, CHHC, AADP 40

PRACTICE 5 **Mood and Food**
By Marita Plozza, HHC 50

PRACTICE 6 **Increase Energy and Live With Vitality**
By Letitia Fowler, CHC, AADP 58

PRACTICE 7 **The Mind/Gut Symbiosis: Finding Super Me**
By Maureen Huntley, CHHC, AADP 69

PRACTICE 8 **Eating for Enjoyment**
By Hannah Heinz, CHHC, AADP 76

PRACTICE 9 **From Heaven to My Plate**
By Christine Marmoy 84

PRACTICE 10 **Sacred Source Eating (Organic, Clean, Real)**
By Fawn MacMichael, CHHC, AADP 92

PRACTICE 11 **Healthy Proteins**
By Tosca Page 100

PRACTICE 12 **Eating With Self-Respect**
By Rachel Miller, CHHC, AAD, CPT, PTA. 108

PRACTICE 13 **The Sacred Kitchen**
By Sarah Mastriani-Levi, CHHC, AADP, RYT. 114

PRACTICE 14 **Love in the Kitchen**
By Cortney Chaite, CHC. 122

PRACTICE 15 **Finding Acceptance with Food Allergies and Intolerances**
By Tracey Camier, CHHC, AADP 130

PRACTICE 16 **Keeping a Balanced Body**
By Michelle Grandy, CHC, AADP, CRICF, RYT 138

PRACTICE 17 **Healthy Sugars**
By Abby Phon, CHHC, AADP, IAHC. 146

PRACTICE 18 **Finding Happiness through Non-judgment**
By Diane Hoch, CHC 154

PRACTICE 19 **The Health Benefits of Being Present**
By Robin Von Schwarz, CHHC, AADP, RYT 164

PRACTICE 20 **Reflection: How Did That Meal Affect Me?**
By Andrea Lambert. 172

PRACTICE 21 **Exploring the Senses**
By Sally Eisenberg, CHC, AADP. 182

PRACTICE 22 **Degrees of Awareness**
By Patti Hedrick, CHHC, AADP 190

PRACTICE 23	**Your Unique Experience**
	By Marika Tomkins *198*

PRACTICE 24	**I Eat to Live a Healthy, Vibrant Life!**
	By Jacqueline Allen *208*

PRACTICE 25	**Culturally Interconnected**
	By Kasie Roads, CHHP, AADP *216*

PRACTICE 26	**Freedom Within**
	By Suzi Pannenbacker, CHHC, AADP *224*

PRACTICE 27	**Unraveling the Fat Myth**
	By Kasia Cumming, CHHC, AADP.................. *232*

PRACTICE 28	**A Legacy of Health**
	By Stephanie Locricchio, CHHC, AADP *240*

PRACTICE 29	**We Are All In This Together**
	By Jennifer Bain Smith, HLC, HC *248*

PRACTICE 30	**Say YES! to Sweets**
	By Sherry Rothwell, RHN *256*

Conclusion 262

Join Our Tribe 264

Gratitude

I want to thank all the co-authors for being so flexible. It could get pretty heated with thirty chefs in the kitchen. However, all the health coaches are so gracious and enthusiastic; it was a pleasure organizing this book for all the busy moms of the world. Let me go on a bit more about the coaches in this book. They are all so full of grace, love, and passion for health, you can hear it in their voices as you read their words. You can also hear their pain, as it resurfaced while sharing their story of triumph with you. Every co-author is infinitely amazing, a pleasure to learn from, and the real deal as an authority on health.

I would like to thank all the moms out there who showed great interest in our second book. The whole project is created for you. Most of the co-authors are moms, so we know how eager you are for some quick, healthy recipes, especially gluten-free, and the support transforming into that all-around positive person you see yourself to be. It is a great honor to provide you with a book full of transformative messages to help you manage your weight, diet, and primary foods. I believe you will find every single co-author an inspiration, as a change agent sharing their truth.

I would like to thank my companion for all his graciousness and support he gave me while compiling this book. My love goes out especially to my children. Through this experience, I have gained the confidence and awareness needed to live as an example—with two feet in front of me, no fear of falling, and receiving the all-encompassing love from God. I know I can be the mom they deserve and the unique woman I am.

I would also like to thank the Institute of Integrative Nutrition for coaching us on the importance of "mindful eating" through our health coaching certification program. Without the valuable knowledge I learned from them, I wouldn't be here now compiling this book for every mom around the world searching for a better way to eat, feel, and live. I also wouldn't have learned the importance of primary foods and how they directly affect our well-being.

Most of all, I would like to thank God for the spirit of love, wisdom, inspiration, and grace through this project, and bringing me the best health coaches to participate in this book. I have never experienced working with so many faithful, inspiring women who live with so much kindness and empathy for others. I will always be grateful for this opportunity, and I look forward to many more in the future. After you learn what amazing possibilities life can bring, your whole being wants nothing less than great!

COMPILED BY **HEATHER EDEN**

Introduction

Have you ever had a negative relationship with food? Maybe you didn't feel good about yourself at one point in your life, and it was expressed through a negative eating style. Were you ever stressed out to the point where you literally "ate" your feelings, starved yourself, or threw up just to feel relief? Maybe it was never any of those scenarios, but you may have felt overwhelmed about finding the right foods to eat and feed your family. It simply could be your eating habits are out of control. Negative feelings of guilt and shame develop through denying or resisting happiness that comes from making good choices—for our bodies as well.

"Cook your way to health" means to find the foods you love and what works for your body. It means you keep cooking those foods over and over again, adding new foods and discovering new flavors, evolving with natural foods until you are feeling great, looking great, and are confident what goes into your body is healing rather than breaking your body down. Healthy cooking is two things: confidence and mindfulness. If you are confident about experimenting with food, you have won half the battle.

"Confident cooks are usually made, not born—this means it's never too late to learn how to achieve a bit of kitchen bliss in your own life. Learning to cook is a lot like learning a sport. The beginning may feel awkward and clumsy, but as you get better, you start to flow and enjoy yourself (Melinda Johnson, MS, RD, health.usnews.com)." You will find confidence when you learn the skills you need to practice making healthy choices, create a healthier kitchen, and save what you learn.

If you really want to know what mindful eating is all about, watch a toddler eat their meal. He or she will slowly chew and feel the texture of the food, in silence, discovering the taste, smell, and look of the food. They decide, willingly, what they like and don't like, naturally, according to their body's responses. One strange or extreme added flavor to food and the child can be turned off without words to say why, making it hard for us moms to understand what they like or dislike. Some days they don't like this and some days they don't like that. It can drive mom crazy. If you're that mom struggling to feed your picky toddler, you are not alone. Two words: grazing trays. This allows them to experiment with a variety of foods, which may or may not please their palate. Also, creativity comes into play with small children and eating. Honestly, it's pretty easy to feed a child. They like natural foods, unless there is an allergy.

Allergies are so common these days—skin rashes, hives, eczema, rosacea, and other countless skin and immune conditions are associated with gluten intolerance (candida). Of course, illnesses also arise from toxins, chemicals, bacteria, parasites, and other germs. However, there is no need to fear. There are many steps to take in order to prevent illnesses.

One major step to prevent illness is a healthy diet. *Balance for Busy Moms—Cook Your Way to Health* is full of quality advice for mom from thirty certified health coaches to help you make the necessary changes for a healthy diet and lifestyle. You deserve the best life possible with your family. This is your go-to resource for healthy, quick, gluten-free meals for those sensitive guts. The recipes go beyond basic understanding of nutrition to preparing superfood meals. Some meals are quick, some of the meals are fun, and some of them are sweet, but most importantly, they are highly nutritious and bursting with color and flavor—remember to eat a rainbow!

Balance for Busy Moms—Cook Your Way to Health is a one-of-a-kind cookbook for moms all around the world. The co-authors are located all around the world, and they each have a past full of hardships, tough decisions to make or something to overcome in order to transform their negative story in a beautiful life, fully expressed.

You're a busy mom. You don't have time to eat unhealthy. You need all the clarity, energy, and vibrancy you can get to raise your children. Your husband, companion, or partner needs you too. They depend on your love as well. How can you give so much if you have little to give?

Loving ourselves first is so important before we can give to others. This has much to do with the way we treat our bodies.

There are many artificial foods and ingredients waiting to destroy you if you let them. Disease is right around the corner with our food system today. Our food system is corrupt, and we can only use our voices to change the situation. Moms have the most powerful voices. We have to push until we see results. But change has to come from the inside first. You can't stand up against Monsanto, and then eat a Big Mac or buy processed foods and GMO produce.

We hope you fully enjoy this cookbook, and keep it always to learn and share with your family and mom friends. Learn the recipes. Try everything! You will build confidence just by doing that. When you read the chapters, notice they are called *practices*, inspired by mindful eating practices. Please understand that mindful eating isn't something you just start doing. You must practice it. This means shutting off the TV, cell phones, and music just to be in a meditative state with yourself and your family. Begin with a prayer of gratitude. Use your senses, chew your food slowly, and feel yourself swallow. You can choose one day out of the week just being together in silence to enjoy the natural foods of the earth that nourish our bodies.

Happy Healing!

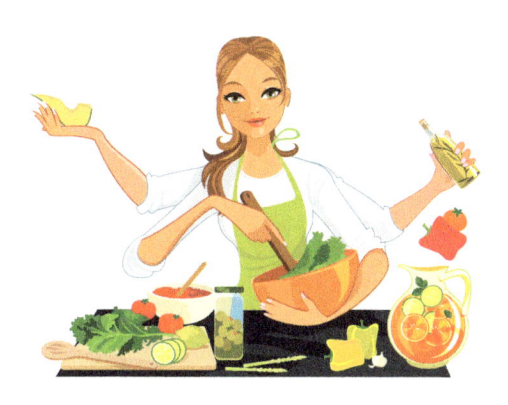

Heather Eden

Heather is an international bestselling author, certified health and lifestyle coach, speaker, trainer, photographer, and healing arts abstract painter.

Heather has a BA in creative writing from LSU, and a certification in health coaching from the Institute of Integrative Nutrition. She is the founder of Complete Wellness Coaching, and *Balance for Busy Moms* and "Balance for Busy Moms Tribe." Heather Eden coaches from the Complete Wellness philosophy of fulfilling twelve areas in life for complete wellness. She also coaches moms on how to overcome stress, unhappiness, toxic energy, and unhealthy habits for a fully expressed, joyful life. Complete wellness means healing mind, body, and spirit through a bio-individual approach, where diet and lifestyle changes become imperative in creating complete positive changes.

- www.heathereden.com
- www.balanceforbusymomstribe.com
- www.facebook.com/balanceforbusymoms
- www.twitter.com/balanceformoms
- www.pinterest.com/heatherluveden

PRACTICE 1

The Power of Choice

By Heather Eden

I am so thankful to have the power of choice. Just think if we had to eat certain things every day without question. Just think if the supply of food was extremely limited. Fortunately, we have many options for food — growing your own, farmers markets or local markets. Some are very obviously wrong, some are difficult to determine, and some are the best and so right for our bodies. Our power of choice gives us freedom, and it empowers us to feel and live with liberation and happiness. This is why being informed about making the right food choices is so important. We have the power—to slowly destroy ourselves or to live with vibrant health, experiencing happiness and joy inside our bodies. The choice is ours. It's not enough to live with the freedom of choice alone. We need to empower ourselves with the knowledge it takes to make the right choices.

If the doctor is telling you something needs to change, and you are sent home with instructions to make a dietary and lifestyle change, you may start to feel overwhelmed—unless you have the knowledge it takes to make these changes. This is where a health coach comes in. Many doctors around the globe are waking up to the necessity of hiring a health coach to help their patients with nutrition and lifestyle. Their schedules are overloaded and they don't have the time to coach every patient.

It is important to understand what works for your unique body and what doesn't—what elevates your blood pressure to unhealthy measures increases your insulin rate in an unhealthy measure, overloads your gut, clots your arteries, congests your intestinal tract and skin, decreases serotonin, erodes your frontal lobe, and creates hormonal imbalances or migraines. Our food choices can cause these effects, or they can support a natural functioning body—for optimum brain, heart, gut, and skin health. You can be an exceptional person with your own internal battle for health, or you can be an exceptional person who lives with optimum health. It's your choice.

Mindful eating is a philosophy of a certain eating practice, which anyone can practice. It's not of any religious affiliation. It simply is eating with the awareness of where your mind, body, and spirit is before, during and after you eat, and using your senses to discover flavor, sensation, response, and texture.

Do you ever notice when your child suddenly doesn't want to eat strawberries? Maybe he or she has a runny nose, and the strawberry is part of the reason why—even fruits and vegetables can cause allergic reactions. This doesn't mean the child will never want a strawberry again. I mean, who can resist strawberries? It just means the body needs a break from it, and it needs something else.

It's 5:00 a.m. and I just had two scrambled eggs cooked in coconut oil, and vegetables sautéed on medium high for two minutes—mushrooms, bell pepper, kale, spinach, and zucchini. I feel great. It sounds like a lot of vegetables, but it really was in proportion to the size of the eggs. This is an example of a food journal. If you want to know how you feel about food and your body, write down how you feel twenty minutes after you eat. Write down what you ate, how it was cooked, and how you feel. Do it for a month, and experience the miraculous things your body will show you.

MY ROAD BACK TO INTUITIVE LIVING

I was raised by parents who took pride in having an organic garden in the backyard and a blackberry vine along the fence. My mother had the "green thumb," as we call it; it means she was good at growing plants and food. Our backyard was tiny, but it was a wonderland of curiosity and life to me as a child. I spent much of my time as a child outside picking berries, honeysuckle, and discovering living things. Those memories are very fond but also faint.

We moved to the suburbs when I was ten, and we didn't have a garden any longer. My parents shopped at the markets close by and trusted in the produce and food. But it was convenient. My mom prepared dinner most evenings, and I usually felt satisfied. The pantry wasn't full of junk food. I did learn some right ways of eating and some wrong ways. However, I was always sick with allergies from dairy, gluten, and processed sugar. It was so bad, I had surgery for a deviated septum at seventeen. But the allergies persisted, of course, because my diet hadn't changed.

My first job at seventeen was a front desk clerk at a gym. It was perfect. I enjoyed working out, swimming, and sitting in the sauna. At eighteen, I was putting women on fitness programs. I had a dream job at eighteen and I didn't even know it. I was good at fitness training, but I didn't know what to eat. My frequent stop after work was Taco Bell. I would leave stuffed and feeling sick, and say to myself, "I will have to work that one off." That was a recurring statement in my head for many years—"Just work it off."

I worked it off for many years, still feeling tired and sick with allergies and fatigue. I visited many doctors for antibiotics through school and college. Even after becoming a mother, and really deciding to make lasting changes to my diet, I still fell ill often and found myself in the ER with my face and body swollen from hives. My nose and head were so congested, a doctor said I would need surgery again. I suppose that was my last straw. I didn't want surgery again. I wanted to find the root cause of my allergic reactions and steer clear from those foods.

I started with milk. I realized that when I consumed dairy, especially milk, I would swell up in my sinus areas. Because milk creates more mucus production, this cause made sense. So I took milk out of my diet. My health improved significantly. However, fatigue, moodiness, and digestive issues continued. I resisted for a long time that it was because of gluten. I did cut down on bread and pasta. But eventually I fell back into my "eating for convenience" mode I was conditioned to practice growing up; and I kept struggling with my health until I realized I felt old, even though I was still young.

When I realized I felt old, and that my happiness came from an antidepressant, I began to dream a better dream. I became aware that what I had set out to do with my life hadn't brought me joy. Therefore, I started searching again for what brought me joy. I began to paint again and experiment with photography. But what I wanted to feel was great! My creativity flowed when I was open to it. But wanting to feel great put me on the path that I am on today.

I became obsessed with nutrition and holistic health. I wanted to find a school to teach me how to eat and live a healthy lifestyle. A year later, I became a certified health coach, and my life changed forever. My allergies decreased and I was able to get off antidepressants and create joy myself. I learned to build confidence in the kitchen and experiment with juicing and home-cooking. Things got a lot better for me once I learned to trust my body cues and follow my bliss.

Mantra: "I am thankful for the power to choose the best foods for my body. "When you eat, be sure to incorporate two things: gut-healthy foods (fermented foods) and superfoods (antioxidant-rich). Cheers to health!

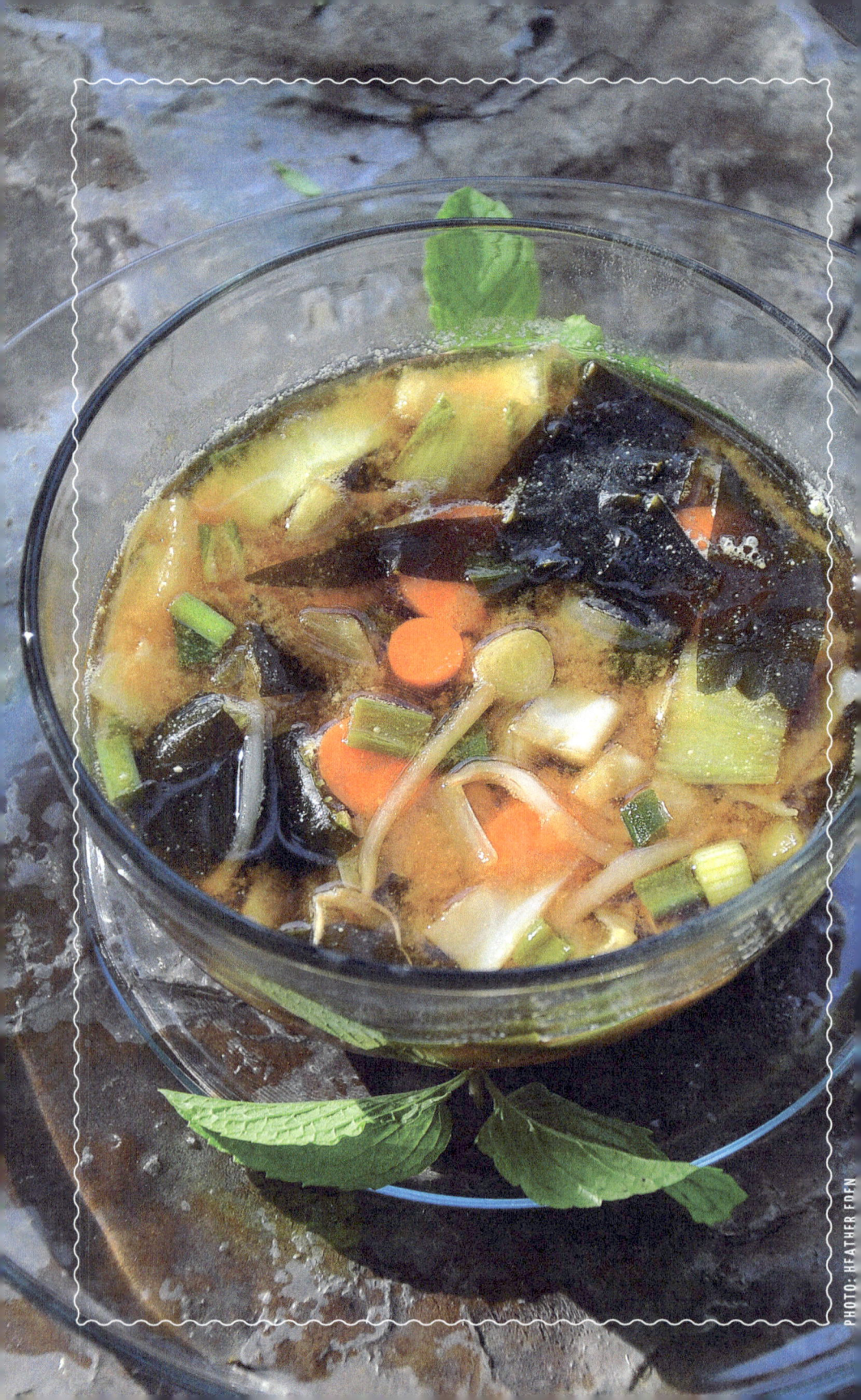

PHOTO: HEATHER EDEN

VEGETABLE MISO SOUP

Ingredients:

- 4 cups spring water
- 1 to 2 tbsp. of red miso paste (taste preference)
- 2 chopped green onions
- 1 chopped carrot
- 1 stalk baby bok choy chopped
- 1/2 cup chopped cabbage
- 1/3 cup of mung bean sprouts
- 1 tbsp. of wakame seaweed
- 1 pinch of cayenne pepper

Directions:

Chop vegetables and put them to the side in a bowl. Bring 4 cups of water to a boil. Add a tablespoon of wakame seaweed, and reduce heat to simmer. Add some hot water to a bowl, and add two tablespoons of miso paste. Mix till it dissolves. Add your vegetables to the water and simmer for 10 minutes. Add the miso and cayenne pepper. Enjoy!

SUPERFOOD RICE PORRIDGE

Ingredients:

- Leftover cooked rice (brown or calrose white)
- 1 tbsp. of hemp seeds
- 1 tbsp. of chia seeds
- 1 tsp. of Maca
- 1 chopped Gala apple
- 1 tbsp. of Goji berries or blueberries
- 1 tsp. of pure maple syrup, coconut nectar, or coconut palm sugar
- 1 to 2 tbsp. of crushed walnuts
- 1/3 tsp. of sea salt

Directions:

Place cooked rice in pot. Fill with water just above the rice. Bring to a boil then simmer for 20 to 25 minutes, or until water is dissolved. Add sea salt, maple syrup, hemp seeds, chia seeds, Maca, crushed walnuts, chopped apple, and blueberries or Goji berries. Stir. Enjoy!

COMPILED BY **HEATHER EDEN**

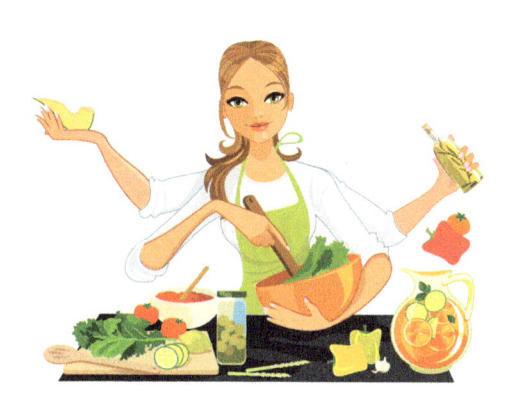

Jennifer Perry, RNFA, CHHC, AADP

Jennifer is a registered nurse first assistant in the operating room, and a certified holistic health coach. Jennifer has an associate's degree in Letters, Arts, and Sciences from Pennsylvania State University, a diploma in nursing from Frankford Hospital School of Nursing, an RNFA certification from Delaware County Community College, and a certificate in holistic health coaching from the Institute for Integrative Nutrition. Jennifer is the creator of Jennifer Perry Holistic Health Coaching and collaborates with physicians in developing programs that will complement their patients' medical treatment, including weight-loss programs, anti-inflammatory diets, and wellness workshops.

- www.jenniferperrycoaching.com
- www.wholebodywholeyou.usana.com
- jperryholisticcoach@gmail.com
- www.facebook.com/JenniferPerryHealthCoaching
- 267-463-7684

BALANCE FOR **BUSY MOMS**

PRACTICE 2

Listening to Our Internal Cues

By Jennifer Perry, RNFA, CHHC, AADP

One late afternoon about seven years ago, I was lying on my couch after a ten-hour shift in the operating room. It was way past dinnertime and my kids hadn't eaten yet. The thought of homework, baths, and the bedtime routine was enough to make me cringe. A friend left me a voicemail asking if I wanted to go to the gym. I put my arm across my face and continued to just lie there. My whole body ached. I'm sure my family and co-workers were sick of hearing about my belly pains. Go to the gym? No way! I didn't even have enough energy to pick my head up. I was thirty-four years old but felt like seventy-four. Something was not right. We all know when there is a glitch in the system, and I knew. The problem was trying to convince the "professionals." Multiple trips to my family physician resulted in orders for lab testing, procedures, and referrals to more specialists. I think I must have seen every medical specialist. I always got the same answer, "Everything looks normal."

I finally sought out a holistic practitioner who tested my nutritional status, hormone balance, and food sensitivities. The tests revealed quite a few food sensitivities and nutritional deficiencies. As soon as I removed those foods from my diet, the abdominal pain and bloating subsided. When my nutritional deficiencies and hormone imbalances were addressed, my energy returned. Although this physician had some medications and supplements to immediately address the problems, I eventually was able to balance almost everything out with FOOD.

I was extremely happy and wanted to share with others this treasure of knowledge I had come upon. I decided to enroll in a holistic health coach certification program at the Institute for Integrative Nutrition. I learned an abundance of information about food from every angle imaginable. I had acquired so much information and all I wanted to do was share! My family was along for the ride, like it or not! They were force-fed many strange concoctions and recipes as I searched for my own style.

Now I see food in a totally different light. It is not just something to quickly calm the hunger pains. Food is nourishing. It gives us energy, helps stabilize our hormones, helps boost our immunity, and even makes us feel warm and cozy. When shopping for food now, it is important to not just view the ingredients according to what tastes good but also look for foods that will support whatever our bodies need. Try to listen to your internal cues. Our bodies tell us what we need, we just have to listen.

When facing bitter cold in the winter and exposure to people suffering with illness, I know it is important to provide myself and my family with foods that are warming and support the immune system. Warm winter soups and stews started with homemade stock, loaded with vitamin-packed root vegetables, and infused with fresh herbs, are a staple in our home in the fall and winter. Roasted vegetables are also extremely tasty and go with any meal. For that occasional sore throat or virus, fresh ginger and lemon tea is excellent for an extra boost of vitamin C and antioxidants. I have to mention my winter standby—homemade chicken soup, a must during cold season. Of course, I make the stock from scratch, and if you never have, I should tell you that it is very easy if done in a crockpot overnight. There is nothing better than waking up to the smell of homemade stock! It will bring you back to the days of coming home from school when Mom had something delicious cooking on the stove!

I can't wait for springtime and the arrival of berries! Jam-packed with antioxidants, these little immune boosters are so yummy we can't keep enough in the house. Berry smoothies, fresh Greek yogurt topped with blackberries, blueberry buckwheat muffins, and strawberry rhubarb crisp are some delicious spring menu options. Spring is also a time when everyone is starting to spend more time outdoors—playing sports, gardening, or fishing. More activity means your body requires more protein and calories. It is especially important if you have active children to keep some healthy protein-packed snacks on hand. My homemade Peanut Butter Protein Bites are easy to make, full of protein and fiber, and small enough to just pop in your mouth. Great for a kid on the go!

Summer meals are by far, my absolute favorite. Garden vegetables can be included in everything from green juices, breakfast frittatas, summer salads, roasted veggie appetizers, and even desserts like zucchini bread and carrot muffins. These foods are very cooling and hydrating to the body in the hot summer months. Speaking of hydration, I was recently turned on to a fun summer drink: fruit and herb infused water. This idea was inspired by hotel spas around the country. It is so easy but looks extremely elegant. Think cucumber, melon, and mint; or strawberry and lime. Good-bye boring bottled water…hello spa water! Wild-caught fish is not only delicious in the summer, but a great source of Omega 3 fatty acids. These healthy fats help our skin look supple, stabilize our hormones, and are natural brain boosters. The children can always use a little brain boosting before they go back to school!

As a nurse, I realize that there are times when medications are needed for immediate problems. As a health coach, however, I encourage listening to our bodies and using nature's gifts to support us on a daily basis. Many of the clients I coach suffer from inflammatory bowel issues and autoimmune disorders. It is important to tune in to our bodies when faced with these conditions. Making home-cooked meals, buying organic, and replacing toxic foods with fresh whole foods are just a few ways we can become the healthiest version of ourselves.

PEANUT BUTTER PROTEIN BITES

These are great little snacks for children who play sports. They are very easy to prepare and the kids will love to help mix the batter and form the balls! I use my high-powered blender to grind the oats into flour, but you can purchase prepared oat flour.

Ingredients:

- 2 cups gluten-free organic oats or 1 1/2 cups gluten-free oat flour
- 1 cup vanilla protein powder (I use Nutrimeal Free)
- 1/2 cup organic peanut butter
- 1 cup unsweetened almond milk
- Dried cherries

Directions:

Using a high-powered blender, grind oats into a fine flour. Add the protein powder. I use a protein blend from USANA called Nutrimeal Free. It is gluten-free, soy-free, dairy-free, and fructose-free. It has a mild vanilla flavor and is lightly sweetened with stevia. Add the peanut butter and half of the almond milk and mix by hand. Continue adding the almond milk in small amounts until the mixture can be formed into a big ball and all of the dry ingredients are well blended. Roll the mixture into 2-inch round balls. Place in individual candy liners or on parchment paper. Place a dried cherry in the middle of each ball for a sweet surprise! Makes approximately two dozen pieces. Keep refrigerated.

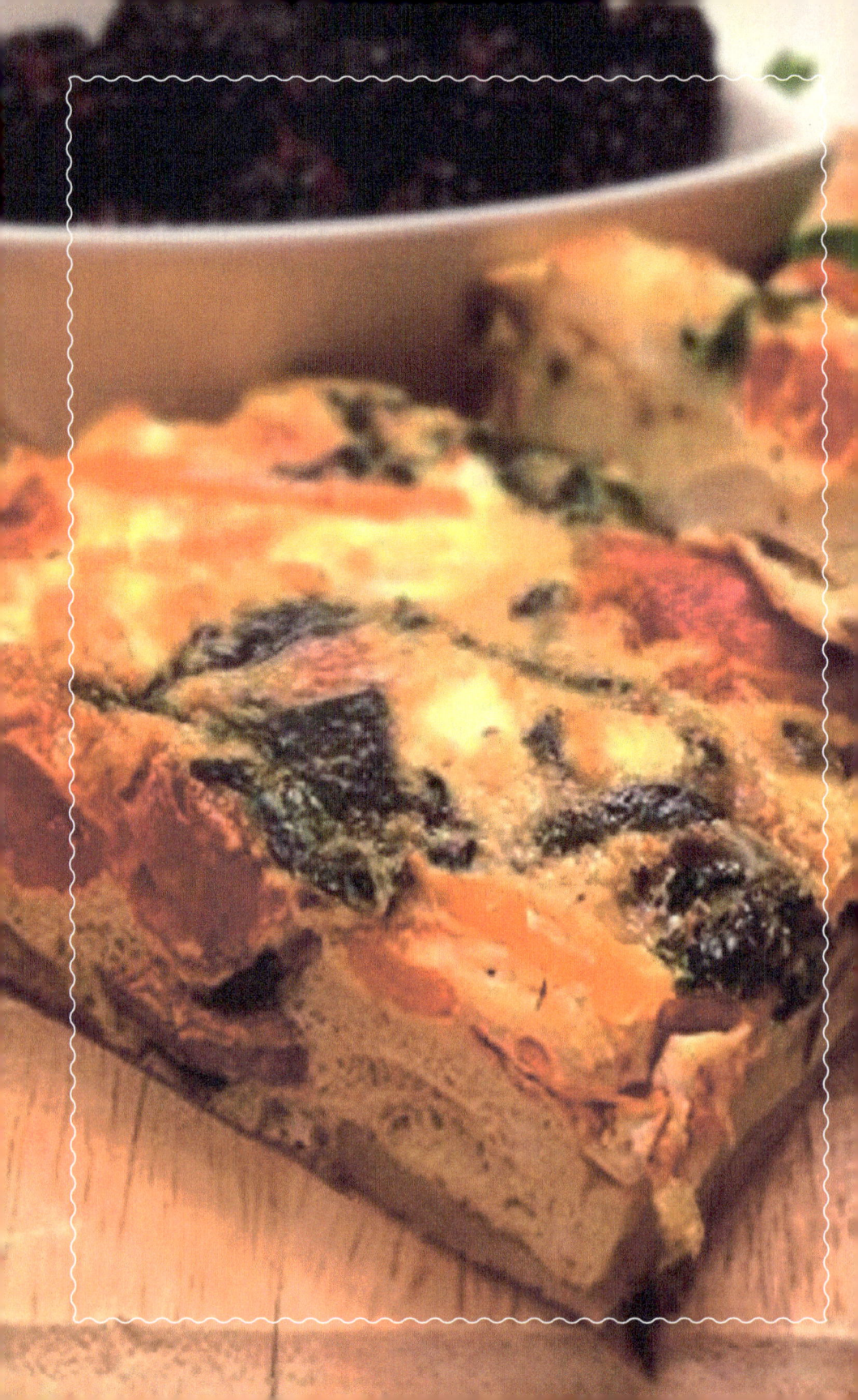

SPINACH AND FETA FRITTATA WITH ROASTED TOMATOES AND PEPPERS

This dish is one of my favorite summer meals. It can be prepared ahead of time, cooled, and cut into squares for easy reheating. Serve with fresh berries for a wholesome breakfast or use it as the main attraction for lunch or dinner.

Ingredients:

- 10 large cage-free eggs
- 3 red skinned potatoes, washed and sliced
- 1 lb. grape tomatoes, halved
- 1 orange bell pepper, sliced
- 1 clove garlic, chopped
- Salt and pepper
- Extra virgin olive oil
- 8 oz. bag of baby spinach leaves
- 1/3 cup plain coconut creamer
- 1 cup feta cheese
- Pinch cayenne pepper, optional

Directions:

Preheat oven to 425 degrees. Coat potatoes with 2 teaspoons EVOO, and arrange evenly on the bottom of a 13x9-inch glass baking dish. Coat tomatoes and bell peppers with 1 tablespoon EVOO, garlic, salt, and pepper and place on separate baking sheet. Place the potatoes and vegetables in oven and roast both at 425 degrees for 15 minutes. Remove from oven and set aside. While the vegetables are roasting, sauté baby spinach with 1 tablespoon EVOO on medium-high heat until just wilted, about 4 minutes. Remove from heat and cool. Reduce oven temperature to 350 degrees. Whisk together the eggs and coconut creamer. Add the cooled tomatoes, peppers, spinach, feta cheese, salt, pepper, and a pinch of cayenne for a slight kick. Pour the egg mixture over the potatoes in the glass pan. Return to oven and bake 1

COMPILED BY **HEATHER EDEN**

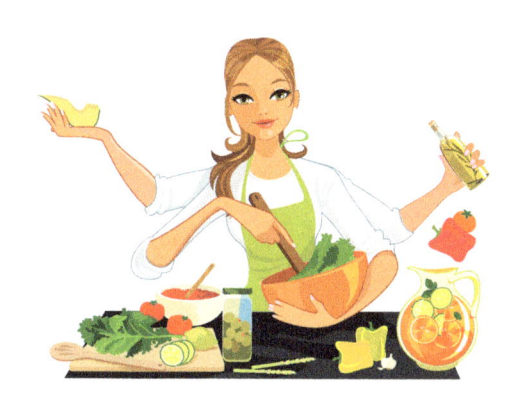

Lisa Bakosi, MS, CHC, AADP

Lisa Bakosi is a certified health and lifestyle coach, speaker, and CEO of Hygea Health & Nutrition, LLC. She works with busy moms to look good, feel great, and raise a healthy family with simple and sustainable diet and lifestyle solutions. She specializes in workplace wellness, cleansing and detox solutions, weight-loss programs, natural living classes, private coaching, and hosts life-changing workshops. Lisa holds a degree in business administration from the University of Denver, an MS degree in communication from Colorado State University, and a certificate from the Institute of Integrative Nutrition.

To receive more than forty natural do-it-yourself cleaning recipes from Lisa, please visit http://eepurl.com/llVdj.

- www.hygealiving.com
- www.twitter.com/HygeaHealthNut
- www.pinterest.com/lisabakosi/boards
- www.facebook.com/HygeaHealthNut
- www.linkedin.com/pub/lisa-bakosi/16/770/52b/
- www.eepurl.com/llVdj

PRACTICE 3

Trust Yourself

By Lisa Bakosi, MS, CHC, AADP

Relationships don't work without trust, do they? I spent fifteen years not trusting my body. The result? Too many years void of self-acceptance, enjoying food, and extra weight that wouldn't budge. I can't get those years back but in sharing my journey, I hope you will learn through my experience.

A DISORDERED BEGINNING...

I learned early that beautiful women diet. I was on three crash diets before I left high school. It wasn't long before my obsession with weight manifested into a full-blown eating disorder.

I remember leaning over a disgusting gas station toilet, black mascara tears streaming down my face with my fingers down my throat, desperately wanting the Oreos I just inhaled out of my body. Eating them meant I would never be thin and beautiful, BUT I wanted to feel free enough to eat whatever I wanted. I was so afraid of my own desires and had lost all hope that my body knew what it was doing.

THE LONG ROAD TO RECOVERY...

What came next were a series of stepping stones in my healing journey—each getting me a teensy bit closer to healthy. Eventually, I realized there was a difference between nourishing my body and counting every calorie. My focus shifted to quality over quantity. It was an epiphany to realize that what I ate directly impacted my mood, cravings, energy, immune system, and skin...not just my weight. I learned some big lessons that I hope will help you learn to trust your beautiful body.

Shift your focus and tune in — Instead of focusing on what you *should* or *should not* eat, try focusing on how different foods and lifestyle choices make you feel. Right now, close your eyes and direct your attention inward. We're so busy that we seldom take inventory of where we are right now. Try this technique focusing on how you feel after you eat a meal. You might notice some interesting correlations.

Figure out what's driving your cravings — Are there certain foods in your diet you can't go without or control yourself with? You might have an intolerance, allergy, or addiction. To uncover what is really driving your craving, do an experiment (AKA: elimination diet) in which you eliminate typically problematic foods from your diet for at least one week and introduce them back one at a time to see how your body responds.

I recommend working with a health coach, but if you want to go it alone— Google it. I created a program to help my clients with this because it's such a game-changer. We've been able to eliminate unwanted pounds, cravings, migraines, unexplained aches, hot flashes, acne, and more.

Eat real food (mostly) — We all know that our body thrives on REAL (one ingredient) food, but when we get used to eating processed foods we lose touch with our instincts and stop craving them. As you eat more nutritious foods, you'll notice the connection between what you eat and how you feel. Pretty soon, you'll crave the good stuff more often, your energy will soar, your skin will look fabulous, your digestion will improve, and so much more.

Don't overthink it — Eat what your body asks for (assuming you're not eating for emotional reasons or due to food allergy/addictions), and stop when you're full. The cues may be subtle and you may have to battle self-imposed food rules at first, but what you eat and how much you eat is a decision best left to your body.

Eat your cake too — Go ahead and indulge your cravings sometimes. Those with a healthy food relationship don't indulge ALL the time but feel like they can. They also savor every single bite. When it stops tasting amazing, they stop eating and don't torture themselves with it after the fact. Indulging is part of life...and should be. Ask yourself how you're going to feel during and after. If it's not a truly satisfying picture—figure out what you might really want or need.

Get and keep your head in a good space — If you're hard on yourself, you're going to have to work against old habits. Negativity will work against you and any goals you have.

Try this:

- Find ways to feel sexy—accentuate your best features.
- Get rid of your scale—seriously, it needs to go.
- Create a power mantra—something simple like, "I trust and listen to my body."
- When you catch yourself saying something negative—stop and say something nice.

Honor your non-food desires — Do you conveniently ignore that little voice inside you asking (shouting) for change? For me, I had to quit a stressful job, pursue my passion, do exercise that didn't hurt, and clean up some emotional baggage. What are you being called to do or let go of?

But I can't eat what I want and not gain weight — Changing your restrictive food relationship is terrifying. You may feel out of control. Once you banish all the rules and truly feel free to eat whatever you want (and you're not dealing with any food addictions), you will naturally choose a healthy, balanced diet. At that point, you will learn to trust your body's desires and enjoy food again. Getting there is the hard part and it will take some doing. Just remember that your body is much smarter than your mind and trust in that.

What to do with guilt — Food guilt happens for two reasons: either you didn't listen to your body in the first place (you're eating for other reasons like rebellion or for comfort) or you don't yet believe that you can trust your desires. If you practice, it will get easier to hear and honor your body's messages. Pretty soon, you'll be rewarded with a healthy, happy body and a calm mind.

The bottom line — You cannot achieve your goals from a place of force or fear, but you CAN easily reach your goals from a calm and happy place filled with enjoyment.

MUFFINS OF STEEL

Yields 24

Ingredients:

- 2 cups steel cut oats
- 1 can coconut milk
- 4 eggs
- 3 tbsp. chia seeds
- 1/2 tsp. salt
- 1/2 tsp. cinnamon
- 1 tsp. pure vanilla extract
- 1/4 cup grade B maple syrup
- Chosen toppings: chopped nuts, dried cranberries, raisins, chocolate chips, frozen fruit, anything

Directions:

Soak oats in water in the fridge overnight. Drain water before baking. If using quick-cooking oats, skip this step. Preheat the oven to 375 degrees. Meanwhile, in a mixing bowl, combine the soaked oats and all other ingredients. It will create a soupy mixture. Line a muffin tray with paper cups. Spray the inside with nonstick spray. Fill the cups 2/3 full. Now customize them by adding your favorite ingredients. Get the family involved in the fun. Fill them to just below the rim of the paper for best results. Bake for approximately 45 minutes or until a toothpick comes out clean. Let them cool. You can eat these warmed up with cream in the morning, cold for a snack, or even dessert. To save time, bake in bulk and freeze them. Enjoy!

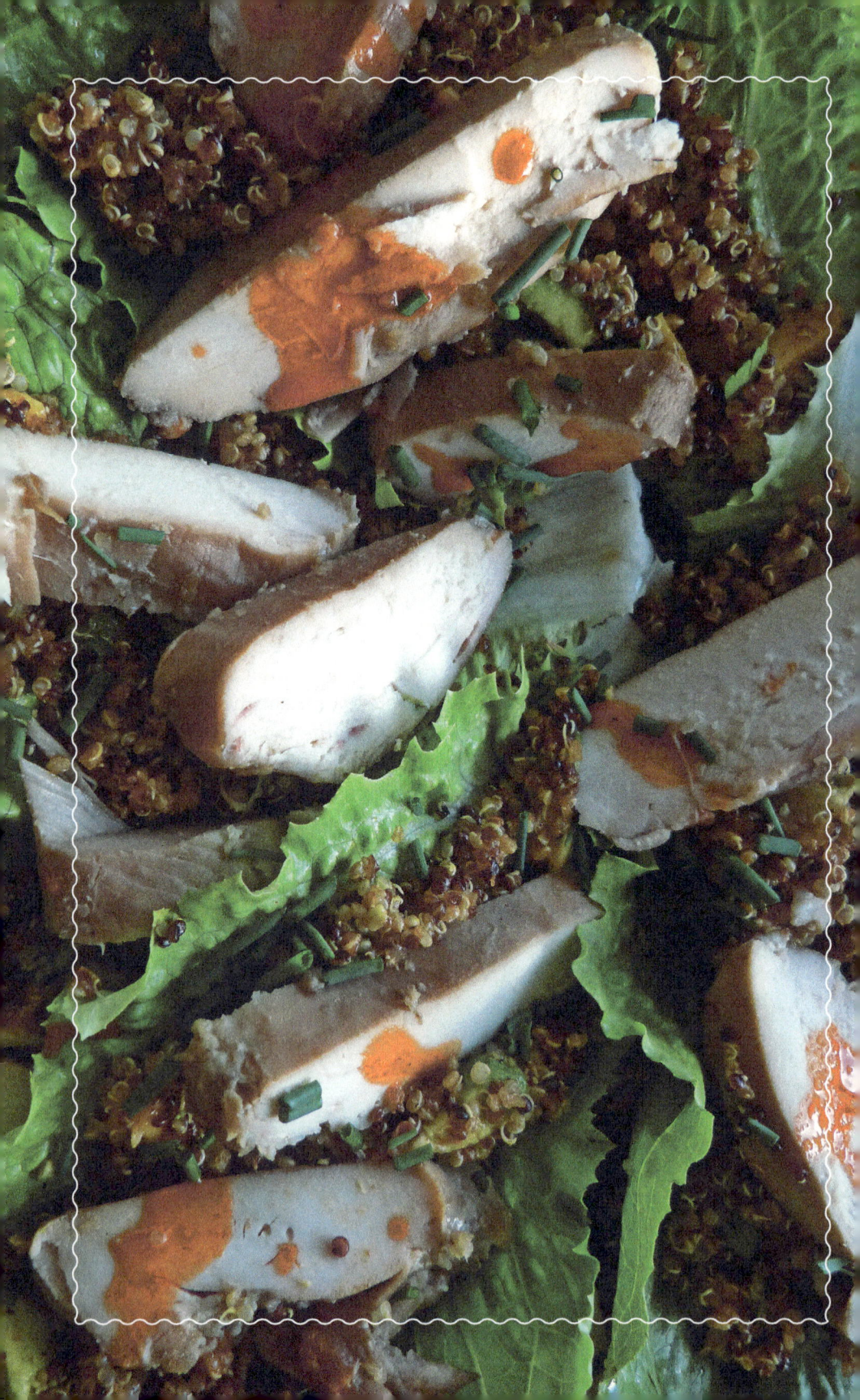

CARIBBEAN CHICKEN AND QUINOA LETTUCE WRAPS

Ingredients:

- 1 cup quinoa
- 2 cups water
- 1 to 2 small mangos, pitted, peeled, and diced
- 1 small can pineapple chunks, diced, juice reserved
- 1 can black beans, rinsed
- 2 cloves of garlic, minced
- Several tbsp. Bragg's Liquid Aminos
- 1 avocado, pitted and diced
- 1/4 cup cilantro, finely chopped
- Juice of 2 limes
- Handful of dried cranberries
- 2 tbsp. olive oil
- 2 tbsp. red wine vinegar
- 2 tsp. honey
- 1 tsp. chili powder
- 1/2 tsp. cumin
- 1/2 tsp. smoked paprika
- 1/2 tsp. sea salt
- Butter lettuce leaves
- 4 chicken breasts
- Hot sauce (optional)

Directions:

In a bowl, cover chicken with juice from the can of pineapple. (Reserve fruit for later.) Add Bragg's Aminos to cover. Add minced garlic. Store in the fridge for at least 2 to 3 hours, until ready to bake. Preheat oven to 350 degrees. Place chicken in a baking dish and cover with foil. Bake for 20 minutes or until done. Let cool and chop into bite-size pieces. While chicken is cooking, bring quinoa and water to boil in a small saucepan. Cover and reduce to simmer for 10 to 15 minutes, until the water has been absorbed. Remove from the heat, and keep covered for another 5 minutes. Fluff with a fork and transfer to a mixing bowl. Let cool. While the quinoa is cooling, prepare the dressing. Whisk lime juice, oil, vinegar, honey, and spices together in a small bowl.

Set aside. Combine quinoa, chicken, mangoes, pineapple, avocado, beans, cranberries, and herbs. Pour dressing over the salad and mix until coated. Scoop the quinoa salad into the lettuce leaves. Add hot sauce and enjoy.

COMPILED BY **HEATHER EDEN**

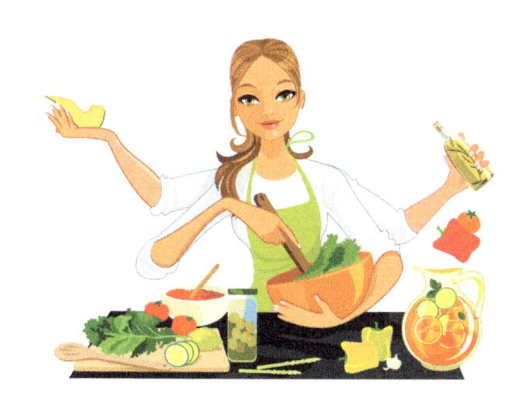

Sarah Mobry, CHC, AADP

In her mission to lose one hundred pounds, Sarah Mobry found that weight management is more than what's printed on a food label. She found a new mission: to help other women enduring the same struggles. Sarah coaches busy moms to release excess weight in her position as a Wellness Mentor. Her clients discover better health, confidence, and balance along the way! Sarah completed holistic programs through the Institute for Integrative Nutrition and University of North Dakota, and recently became a certified personal trainer.

🏠 www.myidwellness.com

PRACTICE 4

Lose the Labels, Lose the Weight

By Sarah Mobry, CHHC, AADP

Weight is an emotionally charged topic—and the feelings it dredges up are usually not positive. Nearly all of us have tried one (or several) of the hundreds of diets on the market. Sometimes they work, sometimes they don't—sometimes they make us feel great, and sometimes we end up miserable. Parents have the added challenge of managing their own weight while also teaching children healthful habits and body confidence. As a weight-loss coach, I see dozens of clients who have yo-yoed through years of weight gains and losses, never quite finding satisfaction or long-term success. For some, it becomes a nagging lifelong struggle.

Most products and services in the weight loss industry have one of two paths: restrict the foods we eat, or utilize supplements, drugs, or surgery to accelerate fat loss. Each book, company, or method promises swift results, near-guaranteed success, and little effort to achieve it. But if it is that simple, why do they all disagree, and why do most dieters fail? Rather than focusing on the standard rhetoric, I'd like us to consider a concept that goes beyond what most weight-loss companies address. By challenging what we have been taught about weight management, we can begin to shift ourselves to a more balanced frame of mind.

ONE SIZE DOES NOT FIT ALL

Many dieters fail to consider that diet books, supplements, and commercial weight-loss programs are more about marketing and sales and less about the individual. They make their money not only convincing consumers that their product is superior to the others, but also that it's a *perfect* fit for the potential customer. The problem is that without appropriate modifications, most diets become unsustainable for the average client. So it's no surprise that after completing a diet program, most people gain the weight back and then some.

Chances are, there's no single way to label the way you will eat for life. Most of my clients base their menus loosely on a style that they enjoy, with modifications for their unique needs. It won't look exactly the same for everyone — so don't base your diet off your skinny friend or the guru you saw on television. When you choose what's right for you and/or your family, consider the many factors that affect your weight loss and maintenance:

Basics: Age, gender, medical history, allergies, and intolerances, etc.

Food Intake: Current eating habits, likes and dislikes, cultural preferences.

Lifestyle: Type of work, activity levels, time available for meal preparation, budget, family dynamics.

Personality: Do you thrive on group or individual programs? With guidance or DIY? With more restrictions or more freedom?

Motivation and Goals: Why do you want to lose weight? When will you know you've succeeded?

Sustainability: After you've reached your goal, can you continue your diet with few adjustments? Can you see yourself eating this way for life?

By making a careful, conscious choice about which foods help you thrive, you establish a foundation for success. Being mindful minimizes the number of times you need to "start over," "get back on the wagon," or struggle through yo-yo diets. Knowing that you chose this for *you* will help minimize your stress (which helps release extra pounds in itself!) and encourage you to continue. Release yourself from the need to confine to what a specific book or weight loss brand tells you, and start making choices based on *your* needs instead of *their* sales pitch.

CHANGE YOUR WORDS, CHANGE YOUR LIFE

How many times have you been told (or told your children) to eat something because it's "good for you"? Did this information give you any desire to eat the food in question? Probably not. From an early age, we develop a subconscious classification of foods being *good* or *bad*. Before long, we begin to see healthy foods, *good* foods, as boring, tasteless, and uncool. *Bad* foods, however, are delicious, indulgent, and all the more tempting since generally they are attractively marketed yet restricted by our parents. This unintentional labeling, harmless as it seems, can lead to significant lifelong changes in the way we see food and ourselves. The war over good and bad foods takes hold in us as children, at younger ages in every generation. I've heard five-year-olds telling their friends candy is bad because it will make them fat. As we get older and learn more about nutrition, it only solidifies these notions, and by the time we are adults, we've created a firm mental connection between *bad* foods and *bad* weight and body image. This insidious mindset invades our whole perception of eating. Bad foods become "cheating" and "naughty." When my new clients have a tough week, they arrive to their session making comments about being punished, expecting an angry lecture just because they had a piece of cake over the weekend. We are adults—whose rules are we following here?

Rather than perpetuate this problem, why not eliminate the battle of good versus evil in your kitchen altogether? After deciding which pattern of eating is right for you, start to think of foods as "always," "sometimes," or "once in a while" foods, rather than simply good or bad. It is a simple way to begin changing your mindset toward food, and in turn, toward yourself.

While you're throwing destructive vocabulary to the curb, add *can't* to the pile. Part of the power of "bad" foods is the notion that they are forbidden. Starting today, change your inner dialogue. Look at the issue honestly: it's not that you *can't* eat a whole pint of ice cream, it's that you *choose not to* because your goals are more important. Choosing not to make "once in a while" foods part of your daily diet puts you back in the driver's seat, where you belong! "Can't" implies that someone else decided for you, that something else has the power. You're a mom, you are powerful, so own it.

AN EMPOWERING MINDSET

Changing the words you use to discuss weight management is a small but important step toward successful, long-term weight loss and maintenance. By empowering yourself in your inner dialogue, you reinforce the idea that you've made a conscious decision to improve your lifestyle and reach for your goals. By using positive terminology and freeing yourself from following one particular diet, you will release yourself from the guilt of not conforming, the stress of following a restrictive plan…and release some pounds in the process!

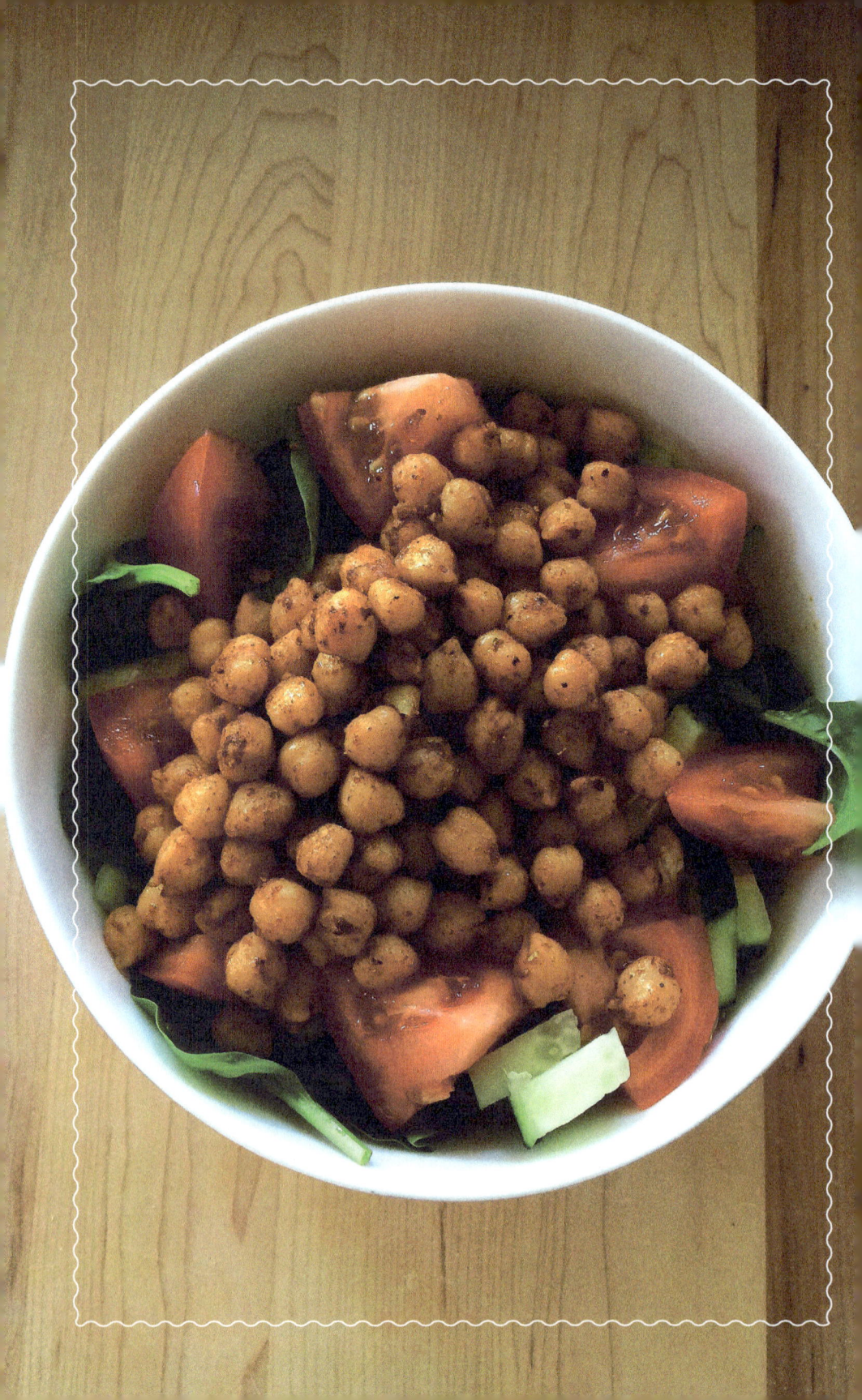

CURRY-SPICED CHICKPEA SALAD WITH YOGURT SAUCE

Serves 2

Salad doesn't have to be boring! Here, chickpeas offer fiber and protein while spicing up your choice of salad mix. Yogurt-based dressing offers a satisfying tang while fresh veggies pack a crunch. Your weight management plan shouldn't be boring—focus on flavor, texture, and variety.

SALAD

Ingredients:

- 3 cups chickpeas
- 1 tbsp. curry powder
- 1/4 tsp. chili powder
- 1/4 tsp. ground cumin
- Pinch of Hungarian paprika
- Dash of cracked pepper and salt
- 3 stalks of fresh cilantro
- 4 cups mixed leafy greens (I recommend spinach and arugula)
- 1/2 red onion, chopped
- 3 Roma tomatoes, chopped
- 1/2 English cucumber, chopped
- Drizzle of your choice of oil

Directions:

Heat oil in a large skillet over medium heat. Add chickpeas and stir; cook 3 minutes. Add curry, chili, cumin, paprika, pepper, and salt, stir again, and cook another 3 to 5 minutes (depending on how toasty you want the chickpeas to be!). Stir in cilantro and set aside (allow the chickpeas to cool slightly, or the greens may wilt). In a salad bowl, place greens, onion, tomatoes, and cucumber. Spread chickpeas over top and serve.

YOGURT SAUCE

Ingredients:

- 1/2 cup plain strained/Greek yogurt

- 3/4 tsp. apple cider vinegar
- Pinch of sea salt
- 1/2 tsp. garlic paste (or similar amount of freshly minced garlic)

Directions:

Whip all ingredients together and serve chilled.

SWEET AND SKINNY SOFT-SERVE

Serves 4

Dieters tend to shy away from dessert, but this one is tasty and won't undo your hard work. I advise my clients to indulge now and then, but to choose treats that still offer some nutrients and not just empty calories. If your blender is not especially powerful, you may need to thaw the bananas first and then put the dessert in the freezer for an hour to firm it up. Otherwise, you can enjoy this right away—it will have the consistency of a soft-serve ice cream.

Ingredients:

- 1 cup nondairy milk
- 3 bananas, frozen
- 1/2 scoop chocolate protein powder
- 2 tbsp. PB2 (powdered peanut butter)
- 1/4 tsp. vanilla extract

Directions:

Place milk, bananas, protein powder, and peanut butter in blender and blend until smooth. Add ice cubes as needed to achieve desired consistency. Refreeze or serve immediately.

BALANCE FOR **BUSY MOMS**

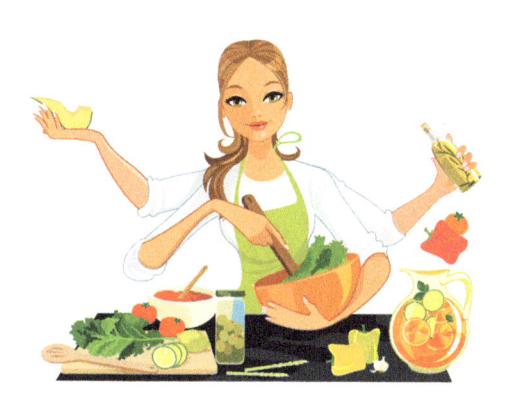

Marita Plozza, HHC

Marita is a devoted mother, wife, and foodie. Her passions include organic gardening, creating gourmet delights in the kitchen, yoga, netball, and raising a sweat at the gym.

Marita believes that the key to happiness and health is creating a life that nourishes you. As a holistic health coach she loves supporting busy women to help them create a balanced lifestyle that nourishes them through whole foods, great relationships, a rewarding career, and energizing exercise. Marita is a graduate of the Institute of Integrative Nutrition; an Essential Oil Expert trained in the AromaTouch technique and is a student of Ayurvedic medicine.

Marita can be reached at:

- www.shakti-flow.com.au
- www.facebook.com/ShaktiFlowHealthWellnessCoaching
- marita@shakti-flow.com.au

PRACTICE 5

Mood and Food

By Marita Plozza, HHC

I have spent the best part of my life contributing. I'm a creative, active spirit. The act of creation in the kitchen is my song, my masterpiece, and my love. I feel a stream pour forth from my heart as I meld and mix my creations. Nourishment from clean organic food made with love. I have the same feelings for my vegetable gardening with the connection to the seasons and the miracles contained therein. My love of nature and the closeness to the seasonal shifts bring me great joy and balance. It has taken some time, lots of learning, and some failure to reach this point.

We have all gone through periods where we consistently eat the wrong types of food. We pay the price with a system that won't cooperate or we are in a daze wondering why our moods are so erratic. The connection is that FOOD affects our MOOD. My son taught me the most about how processed food could manipulate our moods. At age three, affected by the preservatives and additives in artificial food, he developed allergies. We began our journey to a wholefood lifestyle while rebuilding his immune system. We all changed our diet, and not only did the allergy symptoms clear up, but my kids were so placid, so happy to play "nicely."

Our moods are affected by many aspects of our lives: the seasons, the moon phases, our own personal cycles, and that of the world as it swings and surges. We feel the effects of solar flares and droughts, storms and wars. As humans, we deal with many fluctuations in our personal journeys, and that of those close to us, all affecting our moods. There is though a constant in our lives and that is what we eat. Nothing has the capacity to affect us on that subtle level day in and day out as our diet does.

Do you agree that we are what we eat? Artificial, GMO-chemical food, processed in a factory that denatures and depletes it, leaves us in a bad mood. If we are malnourished, how can we be even-tempered and calm?

Your children are largely reliant on you for the food in the house. Your role is one of an educator. You have a certain power or credit in what they eat. If you choose whole foods, unrefined, organic, and in-season, you are essentially giving them the power to grow into happy, grounded, and informed humans. The benefit is your family will get along better, they will develop well, be strong in spirit, and immune to the bugs.

Living in the modern age where we have so much choice, we often feel we have none. Ironically, we feel we must behave or look a certain way. For many, it is now our health that is top priority—not our jean size. In my search for the most common sense proven method, that doesn't require my family to squeeze into a "diet," I came into the ancient Indian method of Ayurveda.

Ayurveda is an ancient way to health, rejuvenation, and longevity. It is founded on the belief that all diseases stem from the digestive system and are either caused by poor digestion of food or by following the wrong diet for your nature (dosha). The system concentrates to a large extent on nutrition and lifestyle.

This ancient system is five thousand years old and is based on two very simple theories of the Five Elements of Theory and the Tridosha Theory.

People and our planet Earth are made of five elements—earth, water, fire, air, and ether—and our unique constitutions (doshas) are combinations of these elements.

Every person falls in one of three doshas (body types):

1. Vata is *air* and *ether*.
2. Pitta is *fire* and *water*.
3. Kapha is *water* and *earth*.

Each person has a dominant dosha, according to their particular body composition, complexion, physical appearance, digestion, and elimination, and of course the way they behave and interact. The system follows the three seasons. Foods eaten during a particular season are to keep you in best health according to the conditions and food available (local, seasonal, and organic). Of course, there is much more to it but in a nutshell, once you know your dosha, you eat according to the balancing foods and the season. You are not just eating for balance physically in Ayurveda, you are eating and living to balance your whole person—mind, body, and spirit.

Essentially, we live by the seasons as per the Ayurvedic lifestyle through wholefood homemade meals with some homegrown and local organic produce. We follow the doshas for each of our systems, knowing this helps keep a balanced approach to eating and health. For example, I am a Pitta (summer) body type, so I can get overheated and irritable if imbalanced. To cool my system, I eat more raw vegetables and fruits, minimizing my intake of meat, most nuts (except almonds), and steer away from chili and pepper, as it's too warming.

If you are a Vata (winter) body type, you would be lean, cool, and dry and would need more warming, nourishing cooked food and heating foods like ginger and chili. The Kapha body type is spring-influenced, so they tend to suffer more phlegm buildup and put on weight easier than the other types. To balance Kapha, it's best to minimize the overall amount of food intake and reduce oily, heavy, and salty foods.

After combining the knowledge from experiments over the years in raw food, vegetarianism, and wholefood living, our choice is Ayurveda. Ayurveda provides us with a whole system where the basis of the belief is to balance and preserve health mentally, physically, and spiritually.

Visit www.chopra.com/ccl/what-is-ayurveda for further information on Ayurveda.

If you were curious to find out your unique dosha or more on Ayurveda, Marita would love to hear from you. She can be reached at www.shakti-flow.com.au or via email marita@shakti-flow.com.au

You can also follow her on Facebook at

https://www.facebook.com/ShaktiFlowHealthWellnessCoaching

Recipes from Marita's kitchen:

These recipes are raw, easy, and delicious.

CHOCOLATE CHIA BLISS

Ingredients:

- 1 cup Medjool dates
- 2 cups almonds (ground in a coffee grinder, or buy almond meal)
- 1/2 cup dried coconut, plus extra for rolling
- 4 tbsp. cacao powder (can substitute 1/2 cocoa)
- 2 tbsp. coconut oil
- 2 tbsp. maple syrup
- 1 tbsp. chia seeds
- Pinch Himalayan salt (optional)

Directions:

First, grind your almonds in a coffee bean grinder and set aside. You can buy almond meal, but fresh ground is best. Put all other ingredients except extra coconut into a high-powered blender or food processor and process, add the almond meal, and bind it all together. Take teaspoon-size amounts, roll into balls, then dip and roll in extra coconut. Keep in airtight container in the freezer.

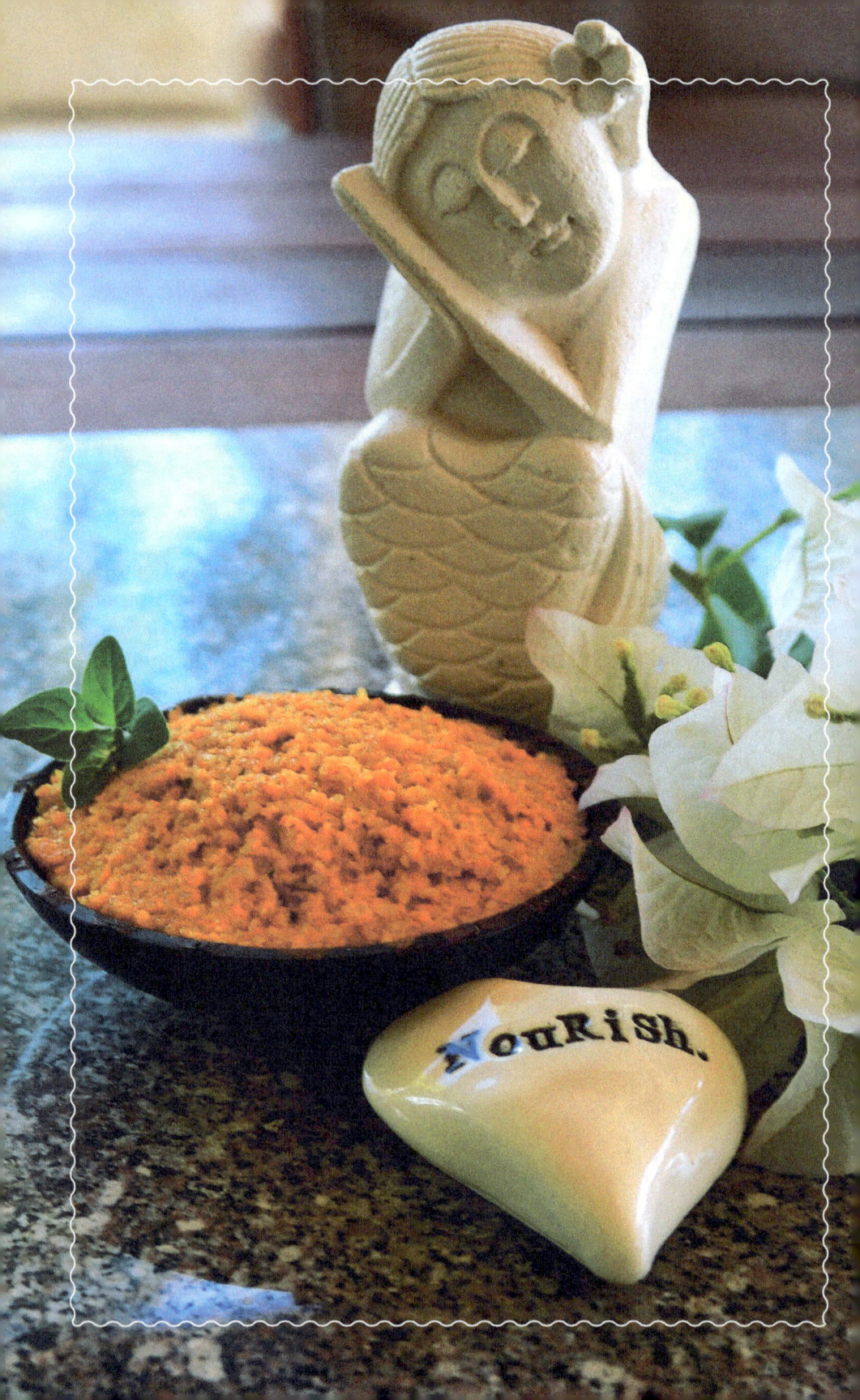

QUICK CARROT DIP

Ingredients:

- 3 large carrots
- 1/4 red onion
- 2 tbsp. oil (olive or coconut)
- 1 cup soaked sunflower seeds
- 1 cup soaked almonds
- 1 or 2 tbsp. tamari (to taste)
- 1/4 tsp. cayenne pepper (optional)
- 1 tsp. cumin
- Juice of 1 lemon
- Fresh oregano & parsley
- Pinch Himalayan salt (optional)

Directions:

Soak your nuts and seeds, as they are easier to digest this way. However, if you don't, the dip will work out just as nice.

Place the nuts and seeds into the food processor or high-speed blender and blend until fine. Scrub and top the carrots then chop into large chunky rounds. Add to blended nuts. Cut onion and add to blender with carrots and blend or process. You may need to use a spatula to push down and get an even consistency. Add the remaining ingredients and blend further till well mixed and smooth.

This dip develops flavor and is always nicer the next day. However, it doesn't retain its bright orange hue. We use this as a dip, a spread, and as raw filling with salad for Nori and rice paper rolls. It can also be molded into patties and cooked in the oven or griller.

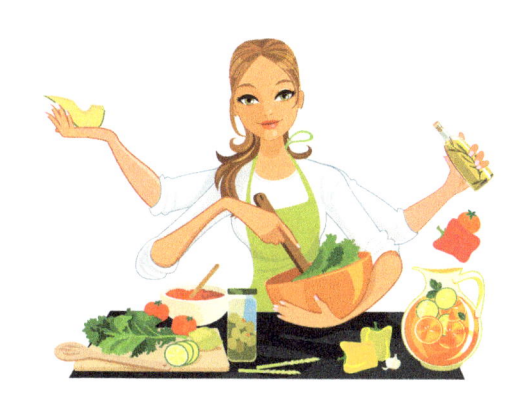

Letitia Fowler, CHC, AADP

Letitia is the founder of Personal Best Health and Wellness. She is a certified health coach, mentoring midlife women that have spent their entire adult lives taking care of other people to make themselves a priority. She helps them embrace a healthy lifestyle so they can optimize their wellbeing, lose weight, and live their life with vitality. Through her nurturing approach, Letitia is able to support clients to make lifestyle changes without turning their world upside down. Letitia is also a certified vision board quest coach, a Reiki practitioner, and has a BS in business from the College of St. Rose.

- www.personalbesthw.com
- www.facebook.com/personalbesthealth
- www.twitter.com/personalbesthw
- www.linkedin.com/in/letitiafowler

PRACTICE 6

Increase Energy and Live With Vitality

By Letitia Fowler, CHC, AADP

Have you ever been hit with life-changing events that took the wind out of your sail? This happened to me several years ago when I was fifty. Less than a year after being diagnosed with stomach cancer, my mom passed away after a brave battle that left her weary. It was especially hard for my daughter and me since we shared a home with my mom and saw her every day. Within weeks of mom's death, my significant other decided to relocate out of state for a new job and the relationship deteriorated. Losing two people I loved so close together hit me hard and my wellbeing suffered.

It took several years of feeding my misery with food and neglecting my health before I woke up and realized I needed to make some changes. Once I made the commitment to being more aware of what I was eating and to incorporate exercise into my routine, I never looked back. I wanted to do what it took to feel invigorated. I wanted to enjoy the rest of my life knowing I was making the best decisions for my body. It was time to make myself a priority now that my daughter no longer needed my focus.

That was the beginning of my thirty-five-pound weight loss, elimination of blood pressure medication, and reduced stress. Having the support of family, friends, and mentors made all the difference during my wellness journey. It was during this journey that I became a certified health coach and learned to listen to my body to optimize my health.

I embrace my healthy lifestyle and enjoy experimenting with new recipes. My energy is at an all-time high.

Let me share with you some lessons I have learned on my wellness journey.

ENERGIZE WITH PROTEIN

Eating protein-rich foods such as eggs, beans, milk, cheese, yogurt, nuts, seeds, whole grains, and dark leafy greens provides your body with a steady source of energy. Breakfast is an important part of a healthy lifestyle and should not be skipped. You may not always feel hungry, but eating breakfast will balance your nutrients and help prevent late night snacking. *By giving your body a consistent schedule, it allows you to maintain sustainable energy.* Avoiding sugary foods for breakfast is crucial in positioning your day for optimal energy, while also helping to prevent cravings throughout the day.

One of the significant changes I have incorporated that has given me more energy is the addition of green smoothies to my morning routine. Green smoothies are most beneficial when made with leafy green vegetables such as kale, spinach, and romaine lettuce. One of the best things about green smoothies is the variety of ingredients you can add to make it pleasing to your own palate. Adding a protein, such as hemp powder, will slow digestion, thus preventing spikes in blood sugar while sustaining energy. An energizing green smoothie that you enjoy is the secret to making it a habit and part of your healthy regimen. Some other nutritious breakfast options include a vegetable omelet. Eggs are a powerful protein source, as well as quinoa porridge or full-fat yogurt with low sugar—"reduced fat" is usually replaced with sugar. By incorporating variety with choices you enjoy and adding nutritious ingredients, you will be more likely to eat breakfast, especially when you notice your increased energy level.

HYDRATE OFTEN

Staying hydrated is also fundamental in maintaining your energy level. Sugary drinks or caffeinated beverages are not ideal for hydration. Drinking filtered water throughout the day will keep all your organs

BALANCE FOR **BUSY MOMS**

functioning at their optimal levels and will not leave you feeling fatigued. Even mild dehydration can cause sleepiness or weakness. *Do not wait to feel thirsty: drink consistently.*

For better digestion, drink water at least thirty minutes before eating. This allows time for the water to enter the cells of your body and hydrate your stomach lining. By optimizing digestion, your body will have more energy for other tasks. Adding lemons, limes, apples, cucumbers, or oranges gives your water some pizzazz and makes it more appealing to drink. Drink half your body weight in ounces. For example: if you weigh 128 pounds, aim for sixty-four ounces or eight cups of water a day. Also, check to see how your body is tolerating the amount of water. Everyone is different, and finding what works for you is the key to feeling energized.

FAST IS NOT ALWAYS BEST

Processed foods can really deplete your energy. The public is bombarded with advertisements of foods that are filled with artificial ingredients containing little nutritious value. Since most of our days are busy with numerous tasks, it is tempting to grab fast food while on the run because it is so accessible. But eating processed food decreases your energy and you end up feeling worse.

Planning ahead helps to prevent the temptations of fast foods. Nuts and fruits are easy to take with you when you are away from home and you can eat them when hunger pains strike. *Making the time to prepare your own meals is essential to maintaining your wellbeing.* When you cook, you know exactly what is in your meals and can prepare them to your own liking. A time-saving strategy is to cook once, eat twice. Enjoy your specially made meal another day or freeze for a later time.

NATURAL SUGAR IS OPTIMAL

Your major energy source is glucose. This is a sugar that is produced from the digestion of carbohydrates from the food you eat. Glucose is absorbed into your blood to give it energy. Insulin is the hormone that retrieves glucose from blood and transfers it to cells where energy is produced. Extra glucose is stored in the liver and muscles for energy between meals, but it can also be converted to fat and stored in fat cells. The body obtains glucose quickest from foods with fructose, thus giving you quick energy and a "sugar high." But this is typically followed by a "crash" and feelings of fatigue. Check food labels for the sugar content. *Choosing slow releasing carbohydrates found in whole grains, vegetables, and fruits will help keep blood sugar steady and give you the consistent energy needed to get through a busy day.*

Enjoy the following recipes, which will energize you with the protein-rich vegetables, beans, and low-sugar sweet potatoes.

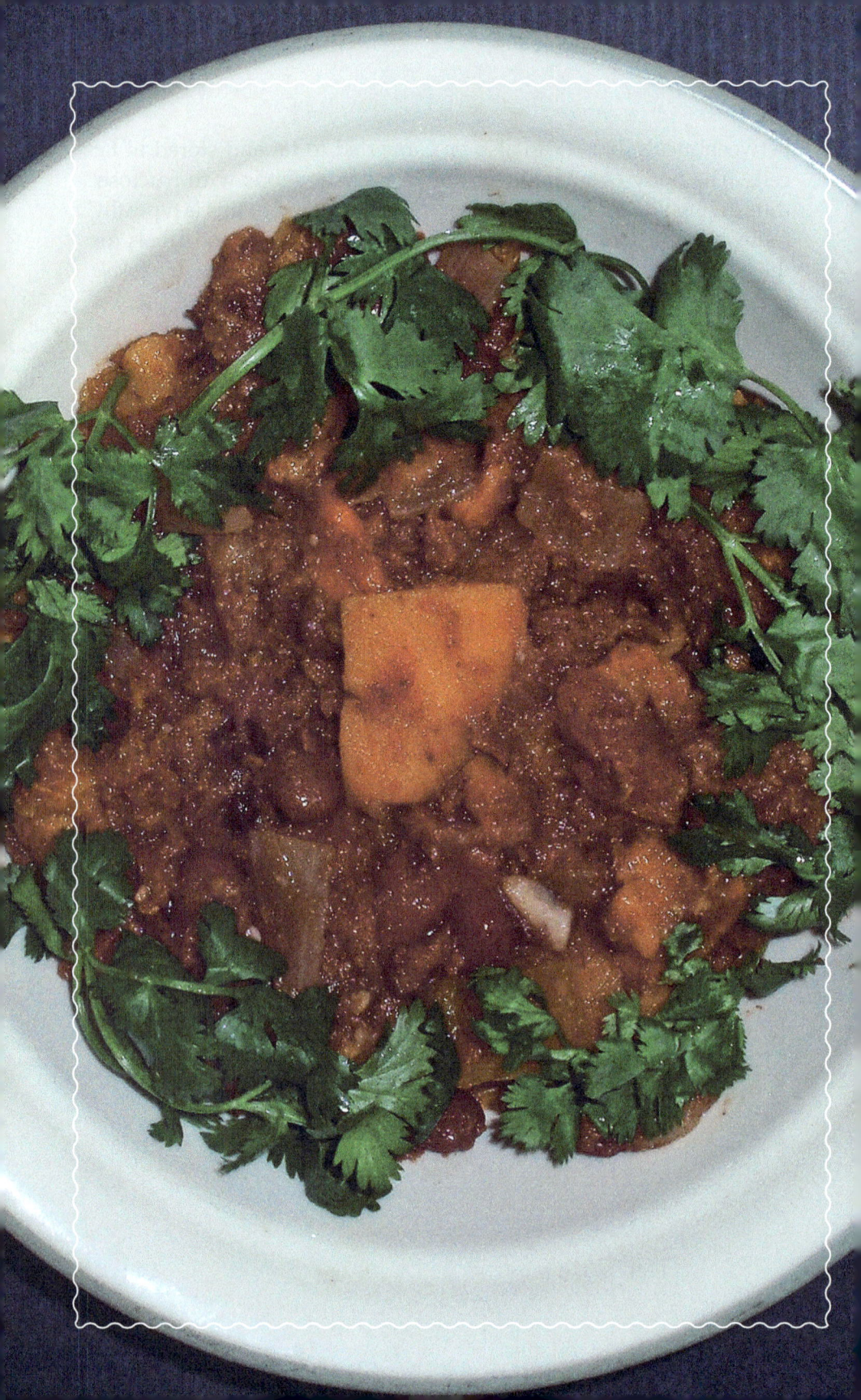

SWEET POTATO AND BEAN CROCKPOT CHILI

Serves approximately 6 to 8

Ingredients:

- 1 tbsp. olive oil
- 1 medium onion, chopped
- 3 peppers, chopped (any combination of red/orange/yellow)
- 2 carrots, grated
- 4 garlic cloves, minced
- 2 tsp. sea salt
- 2 large sweet potatoes, peeled and cut into 1/2 inch cubes
- 2 (15 oz.) cans of diced tomatoes
- 1 (8 oz.) can of tomato sauce
- 1 (15 oz.) can of black beans, rinsed and drained
- 1 (15 oz.) can of red kidney beans, rinsed and drained
- 1 tsp. cumin
- 1 tbsp. chili powder (to taste)
- 1 tbsp. cocoa powder or raw cacao

Optional:

- 1 diced fresh jalapeno
- 1/2 tsp. red pepper flakes

Toppings:

Dollop of Greek yogurt/chopped cilantro

All cans should be BPA-free or use glass jars (Muir Glen Organic brand is BPA-free).

Use organic ingredients wherever possible.

Directions:

Heat olive oil in a pan and sauté onion, garlic, and peppers until soft, approximately 5 minutes. Add mixture and remaining ingredients to the slow cooker and cook on low for approximately 5 to 6 hours. Check to see if sweet potatoes are cooked. Serve over brown rice. Top with cilantro and yogurt just before serving, if desired.

VEGGIE QUINOA STIR FRY

Serves approximately 4

Ingredients:

QUINOA

- 1 cup quinoa
- 2 cups water or vegetable stock
- 1 garlic clove, minced

STIR FRY SAUCE

- 1/4 cup organic brown rice vinegar
- 1/2 cup organic low sodium gluten-free tamari
- 1 garlic clove, minced
- 1 tsp. fresh ginger, minced
- 1 tbsp. organic pure maple syrup
- 1 tbsp. sesame seeds

VEGGIE STIR FRY

- 2 tbsp. coconut oil
- 1 small white onion, chopped
- 2 garlic cloves, minced
- 2 tsp. fresh ginger, minced
- 5 cups of assorted chopped vegetables (Costco sells frozen organic vegetables)
- Pea pod sprouts (optional)

Directions:

Combine the quinoa, garlic, and liquid in a medium pot over high heat. Bring to a boil. Turn heat to medium-low, cover, and cook for 15 to 20 minutes. Let cool for 5 minutes. Quinoa is cooked when each grain is translucent, white germ is visible, and liquid is absorbed. Combine all the ingredients for the stir fry sauce in a small saucepan and simmer for 15 minutes.

In a large pan, heat coconut oil and add garlic, ginger, and onion. Simmer until brown. Add a little more oil if needed and add in all of the vegetables (except sprouts). Mix thoroughly and cover the pan so the vegetables can steam. Cook until vegetables are tender but crisp.

Add stir fry sauce to veggie mixture and heat through.

Serve in a bowl with quinoa and top with pea pod sprouts.

Use organic ingredients wherever possible.

COMPILED BY **HEATHER EDEN**

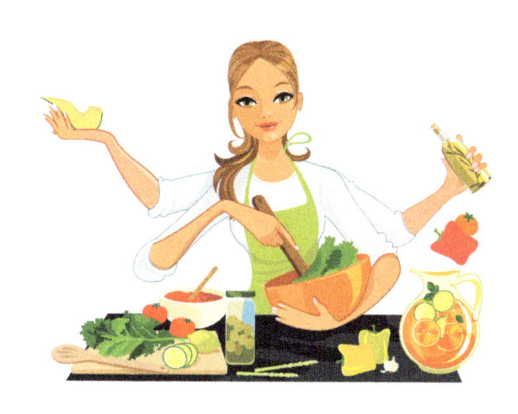

Maureen Huntley, CHHC, AADP

Maureen Huntley, CHHC, AADP is the creator and founder of Mo Green Juice DBA, Vital Health for Life, LLC. Mo Green Juice can be found presently in the NJ/NY region, farmers markets, Whole Foods and growing!

Maureen a graduate of DePaul University, the Institute of Integrative Nutrition and Teachers College at Columbia University is certified in Reflexology, Reiki, EFT, Law of Attraction and as Vegan/Raw/Living Foods Chef.

- www.mogreenjuice.com
- www.facebook.com/MoGreenJuice
- mo@mogreenjuice.com
- www.thefamilybalancingact.com
- www.maureenhuntley.com
- www.vitalhealthforlife.com

COMPILED BY **HEATHER EDEN**

PRACTICE 7

The Mind/Gut Symbiosis: Finding Super Me

By *Maureen Huntley, CHHC, AADP*

I am superwoman! Yes, and supermom, wife, daughter, sister, friend, neighbor, radio show host, entrepreneur, and volunteer. Even as I, superwoman, collapsed on the kitchen floor, writhing in pain that was beyond anything I'd ever experienced during childbirth, superwoman tried to summon super perfectionist, but SUPER SPENT showed up. While this immense pain ran up and down my spine as my lower back cramped tighter than a drum, I worried how I could still take care of everything I signed up for. In a moment's flash, I realized that I had lost me. What was left was a shadow of a woman who thought she could do it all.

As I spent the following weeks in bed sleeping, praying, daydreaming, crying, and giving up, my family—my husband Paul and our four kids—were headed off to Mexico, without me. It had been planned for six months and was to be our first family vacation in four years. Of course, as supermom I had to let them go. What else could I do? I'm supermom and wife! It was paid for and I could take care of myself, sort of. With my army of friends, I could. My gut was turned upside down and my mind was swirling in confusion.

Lying in bed missing my brood, with pillows propped all around my body, I kept trying to call the Hospital for Special Surgery in New York City. I was told to set up an appointment for my surgery as soon as possible, but no matter how often I tried to call I couldn't get through. The lines were busy, I was told to call back, or there was yet more missing paperwork to fill out. No matter what I did to get an appointment, it just wasn't working out. Then I got a call from a chiropractor I had contacted out of desperation. He had told me that he had reviewed my MRI and he, too, believed that I needed surgery. Then he asked me if I had considered looking into other holistic alternatives first. I tried to muster up the nerve to tell him that's what my business and life's passion is—holistic health and wellness. I blurted out that I'm a holistic health coach, raw/vegan chef, law of attraction coach, and Reiki master. I continued, telling him that I work with moms to empower them to take care of themselves first and then they can hold the energy for their family. It starts with mom taking care of mom.

As I hung up the phone, a huge voice that had been silenced for way too long burst forth from my chest that screamed: ENOUGH!!!! SUPER ME showed up. "I know what I need to do. I know this stuff. Why am I not listening to my gut feelings? What on earth has been going on in my mind? Why aren't they working together to help me?!"

Grateful as I was for my situation, it was a hard lesson to learn. This manifestation of what I wasn't intending for myself showed up, and well, pull the legs out from underneath me.

What I did next, from my bed, changed everything. I started with water and journeyed to green juice.

I drank loads and loads of water. I'd get up to crawl to the bathroom while trying to control my bladder. Exercising consisted of tightening my buttocks and releasing. That I did for about three hours a day, on and off. Then slight leg lifts and deep breaths became the start to every hour. As I crawled this path back to me, I became clearer. What was going on in my mind showed up in my gut. What I felt it in my gut, swirled around in my mind. Clarity was scarce and confusion was prevalent. What I had allowed to take up residence in my mind was coming from my gut and vice versa.

Got a gut feeling something's not right? Follow it! I thought I was, but I chose to override it and I paid for it. What was going into my gut was also going into my mind: junk food, toxic drinks, TV, news, pop culture, thoughts, feelings, self-respect, and love. Then add in gluten and sugar—the stuff my engine ran on.

We ingest everything. We are what we eat, think, do, and absorb.

This has become my mantra: What is ingested in the body, mind, and spirit show's up in the body, mind, and spirit. Go as green and clean as you possibly can. It starts with you, not with your family—but they are watching you closely. Do it for yourself first and miracles will happen.

So, you think that you already get enough green vegetables in your diet?! It's just the kids or your husband that don't get enough. Really?! The truth be told, most all of us definitely do not eat enough salads or vegetables to get the incredible health benefits that comes in leafy greens. Even those who say they eat their veggies at every meal (including breakfast) don't get enough greens in. Know how you know? The answer is in the toilet. Yes, the toilet. I bet you never thought you'd be reading this in a cookbook! If you're not going to the bathroom and releasing what you've put between the cheeks on your face through to the cheeks on the backend, you're not getting enough greens.

The end. Excuse the pun.

Now, as the owner and CEO of Mo Green Juice at Vital Health for Life, LLC, I'm still working on it. It's not perfect, because I'm not perfect. I'm perfectly happy and settled being imperfect, because I'm only human. I have walked the path, over and over again, learning to respect the green veggie! There are days that I don't eat my greens at all or drink enough water, but now when my gut speaks to me, I listen. I mind my mind in the process. Yes, I'm still doing the super person thing, but with more awareness that comes with age, greens, self-love, and respect.

The following are two recipes that I love, using mo' greens. My hope and wish for you is that it doesn't take a big life event to get you to take better care of yourself. If it does, you will be better than OK if you pay attention to how your gut and mind work together, because the answer will show up between the cheeks.

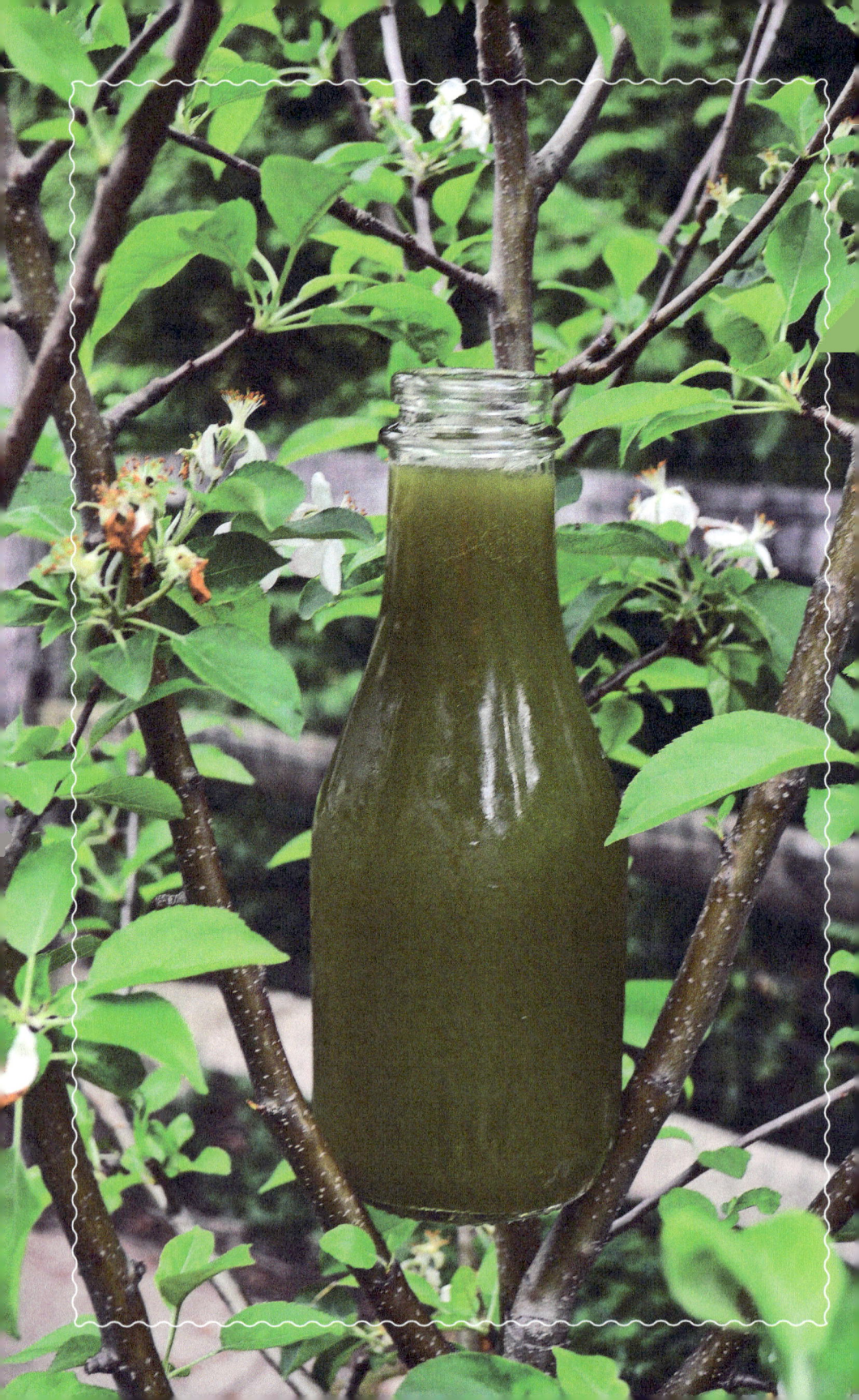

MO' GREENS SALAD

Ingredients:

- 2 bunches of kale
- 1/2 cup arugula
- 1/2 cup spinach
- 1/4 cup pecans or walnuts, chopped
- 1/4 cup raisins (presoaked in water for 30 minutes)
- 2 tbsp. cold pressed olive oil
- Juice of 1 lemon (about 2 tbsp.)
- 1 tbsp. raw honey (optional)
- 1/2 tsp. Celtic sea salt

Directions:

De-stem the kale. Rip or chop leaves crosswise into small pieces. Place chopped leaves into a mixing bowl and massage with the olive oil, lemon juice, and salt, working with your hands until the leaves are wilted and well-coated in the mixture. Add in the honey, pecans (or walnuts), and raisins, blending well to combine. Set aside for 30 minutes or more to marinate. Add in arugula and spinach, and toss. Eat as a salad or as a sandwich or wrap it up in a Nori sheet!

Enjoy!

BALANCE FOR **BUSY MOMS**

CHEEK TO CHEEK: CLEAN GREEN JUICY JUICE

Serves approximately 2 to 4

Ingredients:

- 6 to 10 leaves green lettuce (romaine, iceberg…green…)
- 2 cucumbers
- 3 leaves kale
- 1/4 bunch of spinach
- 2 small Granny Smith or Gala apples
- 3/4 piece of ginger
- 1 celery stalk w/leaves
- Sliver of red and green pepper
- Handful of parsley
- 1 orange and/or large lemon, peeled

(Add a dash a Braggs Raw Apple Cider Vinegar for health benefits with "zing"!)

Directions:

Juice all together for a power-packed, cheek to cheek, clean green juicy juice.

In the end, but not yet to the finish line, the next MRI I had showed no signs of bulging or herniated discs. I know I healed myself by being super to me, for me.

Take a deep breath and know that you are not alone.

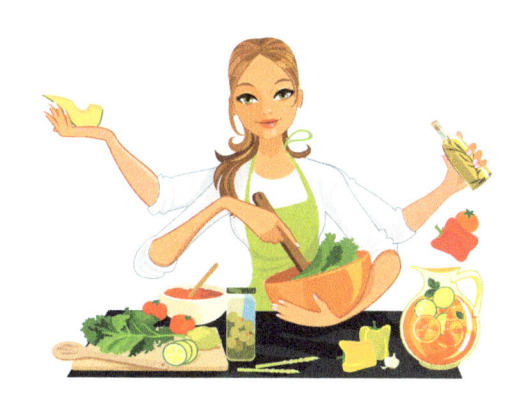

Hannah Heinz, CHHC, AADP

Hannah Heinz is a certified holistic health practitioner and is a graduate of the Institute for Integrative Nutrition, the world's largest nutrition school. Studying at Escoffier Online International Culinary Academy, Hannah is on her way to becoming a professional chef and is enjoying specializing in French cuisine.

With plenty of culinary adventures to share with fellow cooking enthusiasts, Hannah is a frequent writer on health and creative cuisine for her blog, *Hannah's Food Journey*, as well as the author of various eBooks and motivational materials.

Whenever she is not in the kitchen, Hannah enjoys performing piano and spending time with her miniature horses.

- www.HannahsFoodJourney.com
- www.facebook.com/HannahsFoodJourney
- www.YouTube.com/HannahsFoodJourney
- www.Twitter.com/HannahsFood
- hannahsfoodjourney@gmail.com

PRACTICE 8

Eating for Enjoyment

By Hannah Heinz, CHHC, AADP

None of us are perfect, so the best we can do is strive for maximized balance by leading a simple life. By simple, I do not mean "boring," but rather not spending energy on unnecessary things. I like the 90/10 rule: 90 percent of the time, eat as much fresh, real food as possible, but at the same time enjoy that piece of chocolate every once in a while. That is the fun 10 percent! By eating wholesome foods 90 percent of the time, you will not feel guilty when you enjoy the 10 percent since it is intentional. Personally, if I try to eat 100 percent raw, real foods, my resolve lasts for a while and I feel amazing, but before long, I crash and splurge on a lot of food I would not normally consume. It is better to plan it out with the 90/10 rule to avoid bingeing and becoming an impulsive eater. I enjoy cooking and eating every kind of food, so it is hard to skip out on home-style traditional dishes. Fortunately, you can take almost any recipe and substitute better options for typical standard ingredients and come up with a much healthier recipe. That is what I have done with brownies. They are not only gluten-free and grain-free—because I substituted cooked black beans for the flour—they also have a minimum amount of sugar in them.

You may think black beans are a strange substitute, just as I did when I first had the idea! Surprisingly, the brownies do not actually taste like beans. The black beans create the correct consistency and perfect amount of body for a rich "chocolaty" brownie. It's not only a great tasting, easy recipe, it also taught me a thing or two about perseverance and determination. I'm sure you can relate to the following story if you have spent much time in the kitchen.

One day, I needed black beans for a Mexican bean dip. Nothing too complicated, right? Well, for me, who had never made black beans before, it was a fairly daunting task. I didn't know exactly what to expect when cooking black beans, much less how to cook them. I asked my mom and sister how they usually cook black beans, and after an explanation from each of them, I had a vague idea of what to do but was unsure about one thing: does the lid go on the pot at the beginning of the cooking time or does it go on while they sit after boiling, before getting cooked a second time? Surely, there could not be that much of a difference! Since my mom and sister were no longer available, I decided to put the lid on at the beginning, turned the stove on, and left the room for an hour. What I did for an hour without so much as another thought about those black beans escapes my mind to this day. I was probably listening to my favorite composer, Mozart, as his pure melodies soared through the roof to the sky.

When I heard the timer go off, I ran toward the kitchen, realizing I'd forgotten about those silly black beans! What I saw what had happened in the kitchen while I was lost in a Mozartian phrase made me stop in my tracks. My only comfort was that I was the only one home to witness the scene of the disaster. As my eyes scanned the room, it was evident there'd been an explosion: a black bean explosion. The lid that had been on the pot was now on the floor, along with a pile of black beans. They were everywhere! All over the stove, floor, counter, and even the ceiling! I'm not sure how black beans got on the kitchen ceiling, but I wasn't going to try to find out. As I cleaned up the mess, which was quite a chore, I promised myself I was *never* going to make black beans again. "If at first you don't succeed, try, try again" was certainly not my motto. I didn't want to clean up black beans again that exploded like popcorn!

Following the black bean incident, whenever I cooked, I found myself using canned beans frequently. It was not until I had the idea for black bean brownies that I dared approach the stove again with a pot of beans in my hands, but only after carefully researching how to cook beans and listening to my mother and sister's directions more carefully. That incident is a lesson I will never forget. Hey, now I can personally say, "If at first you don't succeed, try, try again!"

You may be asking yourself, "So, how do you cook beans?" Good question! Many people cook them on the stove. I like to cook them slow and steady. When they are cooked on the stove, it's natural to turn up the heat so they get done faster. That roughens the outside of the bean and then the bean doesn't get done on the inside. I like to let them soak overnight, which lets them absorb the water and cook better, and then cook them in a crockpot.

1. Pull out your crockpot and measure your beans, then cover them with about three times as much water.

2. After letting them soak overnight, drain and rinse them.

3. Stick them right back in the crockpot with plenty of water covering them. Don't worry about getting the perfect amount of water. More is better because you can just drain off the extra. Then you know they will not go dry with too little water.

4. Let them cook for a few hours. I think beans tend to cook really well this way. The stove method tends to roughen them up a little because the water is moving and the stove is a higher heat than the crockpot. This way you can let your beans cook all afternoon while you do other things.

COMPILED BY **HEATHER EDEN**

CHOLULA® HONEY MUSTARD DRESSING

Yields 1 1/2 cups

If you are looking for an easy versatile dressing, Cholula Honey Mustard Dressing is perfect for you! I use this dressing many ways. My favorite way to use it is on a southwestern salad with romaine lettuce and a colorful mix of bell peppers, onion, avocado, and cilantro. You can also cut up some veggies and use it as a dip or marinate chicken with it. Put it on a grass-fed burger for a little kick. Dress a pasta salad with it for flair. Share your ideas on how you have used this dressing on the *Hannah's Food Journey* Facebook page.

Ingredients:

- 1/2 cup honey
- 3/4 cup grapeseed oil (grapeseed oil is my favorite for this dressing, but you can use other oils)
- 3 tbsp. Cholula® brand hot sauce
- 1/4 cup mustard

Directions:

To make dressing, combine all ingredients in a blender or jar and blend or shake until smooth. This recipe is great for children to help out with. It is easy for them to help by measuring the ingredients into a Ball® wide-mouth canning jar (quart size) and shaking the jar. You can change up the amount of Cholula hot sauce in the dressing for more or less of a kick. Serve the dressing chilled for best taste.

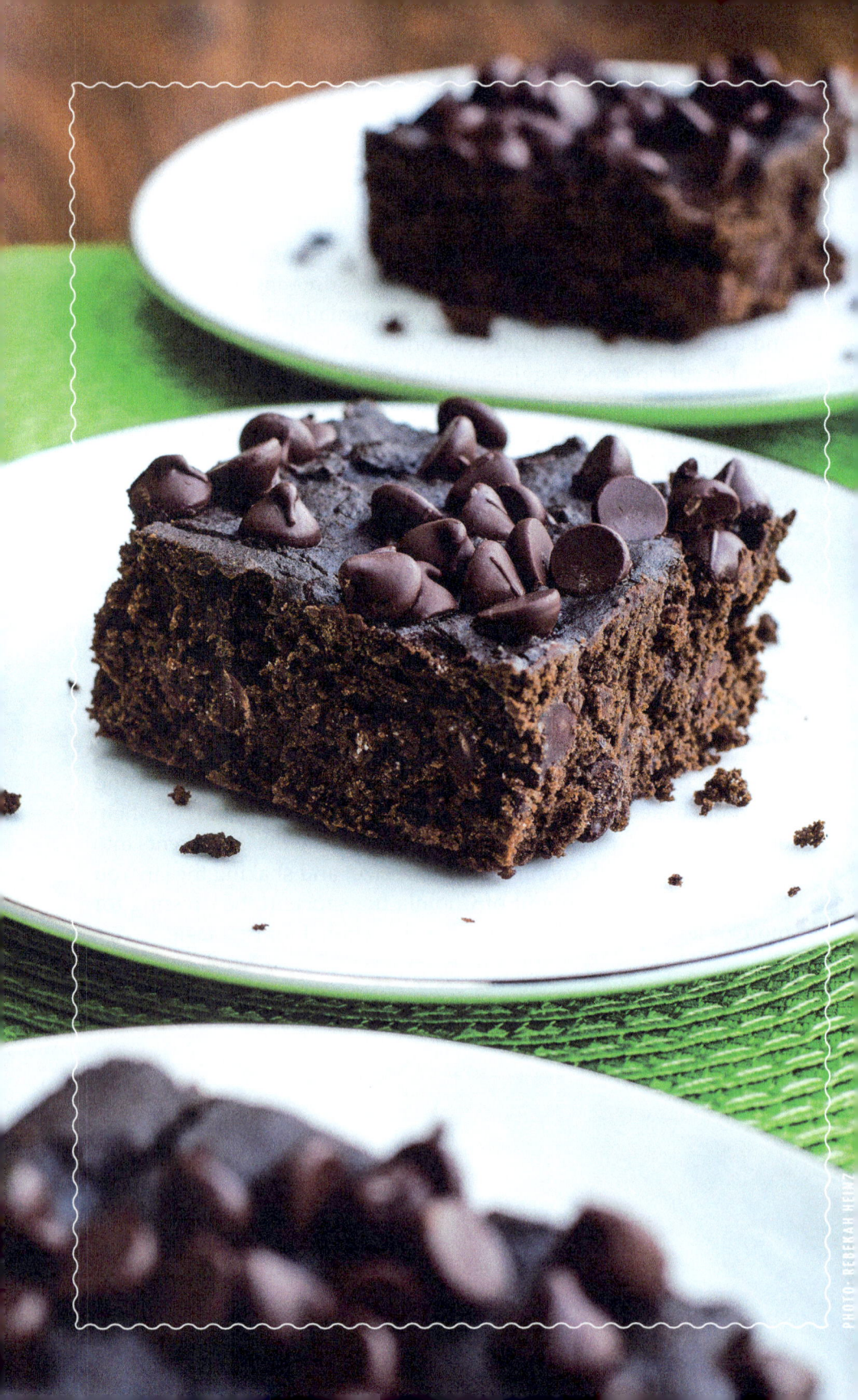

BLACK BEAN BROWNIES

Yields one 9x9-inch pan

This recipe is not only super easy, it is Supercalifragilisticexpialidocious! You would never know from the taste that there are black beans in them. They are super moist and chocolaty. You will find yourself making these brownies time and time again. They will not let you down as long as you don't cook the beans with a lid!

Ingredients:

- 1 3/4 cups cooked, rinsed and drained black beans or 1 (14 oz.) can organic black beans, rinsed and drained
- Large eggs
- 1/2 cup cocoa powder
- 2/3 cup xylitol or sugar
- 1/2 tsp. grapeseed oil
- 1 tbsp. whole milk or milk alternative
- 1 tsp. balsamic vinegar
- 1/2 tsp. baking powder
- 1/2 tsp. baking soda
- 1/2 tsp. coffee grounds
- 3/4 cup dark chocolate chips

Directions:

Preheat the oven to 350 degrees. Grease a nonstick 9x9-inch square baking pan with grapeseed oil or cooking spray. Blend together all ingredients except the chocolate chips in the blender until smooth and pour into a bowl. Fold in 1/2 cup chocolate chips until combined. Pour the brownie batter into the prepared pan. Sprinkle or creatively draw a unique pattern with the remaining chocolate chips over the top of the brownies. Bake the brownies until a toothpick comes out clean, about 20 to 25 minutes. The beans will dry out if they are overcooked, so monitor the time carefully. Allow brownies to cool completely before cutting into squares.

Hannah Heinz

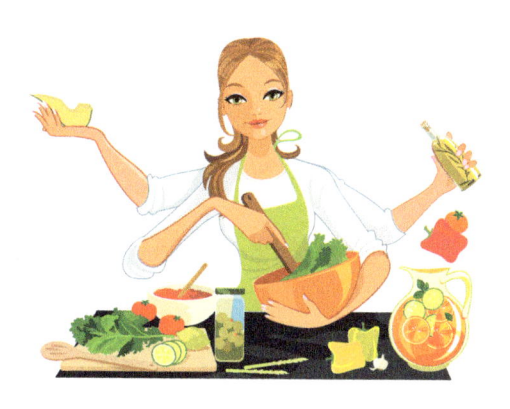

Christine Marmoy

Christine Marmoy is a marketing maverick, author of the bestselling book, *These Dreams are Made for Walking!* and the compiler of two bestselling anthologies, *Success in (High) Heels* and *Hot Mama in (High) Heels*. She works with women all over the world who are eager to become visible on the global market. She finally merged her two passions for marketing and books into a brand new hybrid publishing solution that she now offers to her clients. This allows them to become instant authorities in their field by publishing their own anthology, cost-free in ninety days.

- www.coachingandsuccess.com
- www.successinhighheels.com
- www.hotmamainhighheels.com
- www.facebook.com/christinemarmoy
- www.facebook.com/coachingandsuccess

PRACTICE 9

From Heaven to My Plate

By Christine Marmoy

Most of us spend the majority of our life trying to figure out what doesn't need to be. We complain about stress while we are the creator of it, and we love it so much that it transpires into everything in our life. For many of us stress = having a lot to do…and we all know that important people have a lot to do, right?

We are born with an internal GPS, designed to help us live life to the fullest, enjoying the best it has to offer, but despite that we dismiss this genuine knowledge, preferring an existence in "autopilot" mode with the detrimental consequences that such a lifestyle may bring.

Unfortunately, we do that until the machine breaks down, until we cannot continue any longer, until change is imposed upon us forcefully and painfully. At least, that is what happened to me.

I've always been 95 percent vegetarian. Coupled with that, I was so proud of being a yoga teacher for years….running 10K on the beach every day. Having danced for eight years, I was in great shape, I was doing great, and I looked great. I had won the right to claim that with tears and sweat. Yet, I was eating a lot of pasta and smoking! I still can't believe that I was calling myself "healthy"—talk about self-denial!

Fast forward ten years. A move to Europe, no more running, no more yoga classes, still some veggies and fruit but very little…worse than the lack of these, I suffered more from the lack of taste. Then I reached that fatalistic moment when my body could no longer cope with my lack of respect—no exercise, no fresh food, tobacco, high stress levels—and you have all the necessary elements to create a human time bomb. I collapsed…literally.

I went from being so-called "healthy" to a wheel chair. After months of going downhill, I literally fell to the floor…with the truth resonating in my ears. I like to say that it was coming directly from the Universe. It kicked me hard because that was the only way it knew I would listen. Did it send me signs? Did it warn me? Of course it did, many times beforehand. Yet my ears were deaf to facing the inevitable truth about my future. The wake-up call was brutal, as powerful as the words I was not prepared to hear! "You have MS…you'll need to take steroids and you must change your plans because you will never be able to achieve your dreams, you are suffering from a debilitating disease!"

OK, so I could cope with changing my plans temporarily, but giving up on my dreams? I was definitely not ready for that, and from the moment I rejected this self-imposed belief, I healed myself. Yes, I actually did.

How did I do it?

Well, I got help. The Universe helped me meet a chiropractor from New York. I live in Spain, so that was odd. To this day, I believe that I walk again thanks to him. Then my neurologist prescribing steroids was another omen. When I realized that the doctors didn't even know if they would work—although scarily enough they all seemed to agree on the side effects this medicine would have on my body—my decision was final. Forget it! I refused to put more toxic substances into my body! I had quit smoking one year before—cold turkey—and right at that moment, I decided that I'd get rid of this disease the same way.

It was a turning point because I decided to find ways to make myself feel better using what the Universe had given me in the first place: my mind, my heart, and my body. I did extensive research about the power of the mind through meditation, the healing of the heart through emotions, and the detoxifying power of our body through food. At the time, I could barely walk. I suffered heavy brain fog and in many instances, I couldn't even speak. This was my daily routine.

Two months later, I was walking on the treadmill again, my brain was functioning almost normally, and my speech was back.

Today, I work out one to two hours a day, I meditate one hour a day, and I get up every day at 4:30 a.m. My business is thriving, and I have reached a new level of contentment in my life, which I never knew could exist.

But all this did not come about just by chance! I had to clear out the canal of communication with the Universe so I could hear it speak to me, so I could be healthy and happy every day.

The answer came directly from Heaven onto my Plate. I studied food and how what we eat actually affects the connection with our higher consciousness, which I like to call the Universe. I became obsessed with cleaning the pathway to a better life. From 95 percent vegetarian, I became 100 percent, and then vegan. Eventually, I stepped into the world of raw food and never looked back. I got the message loud and clear…if I was the creator of the disease, then I could very well be the healer. From this thought I'd allowed into my head, the emotions I accepted to feel, and the food I voluntarily put into my body, I had full control.

I quit pasta "cold turkey," I stopped eating bread, and everything that contained chemicals was no longer welcome in my kitchen. The effect of healthy eating became apparent in a week. The fast results became a motivator because they proved to me that I was on the right track. Interestingly enough I realized that quitting bad food, like white pasta, was actually not that difficult. As with every change I had made in my life, once the decision was made, the rest followed as completely natural. While I was still cooking pasta for the kids, it never bothered or tempted me. I felt so much better that my brain was reacting differently without me having to consciously make an effort.

When you think about it, I went through massive changes, I really flipped my life around 180 degrees, and it was all orchestrated through Divine Intention. For the first time in my life, I allowed my body to tell me what it needed. To this day, I never know what I'm going to eat. I eat every two hours and my body is the chef. My daily diet is usually a banana in the morning, a plant-based protein shake with almond milk after my workout, homemade hummus, a delicious salad, some carrots and cucumber with almond dip, then a little soup…and I finish my day with another protein shake right before bedtime. This shake allows me to cut out my sugar craving and sleep better.

Then something else occurred. Witnessing my miraculous recovery and how great I felt, my husband decided that it wouldn't hurt to give it a try. He lost the 10 kg he wanted to. Now he works out every day and feels so much better. And my daughter Camille has joined our Family Health Club.

I'm still putting the intention forward that my five-year-old boy, Mathys, may one day decide to give veggies and fruit a chance.

Healthy eating doesn't mean that you can't eat tasty treats and comforting food. It's all about the quality of the ingredients you use and steering clear of bad fats and chemicals. And to prove my point, I decided to share these bestsellers in my household with you. I hope you'll try them and enjoy them. They are easy and quick to prepare!

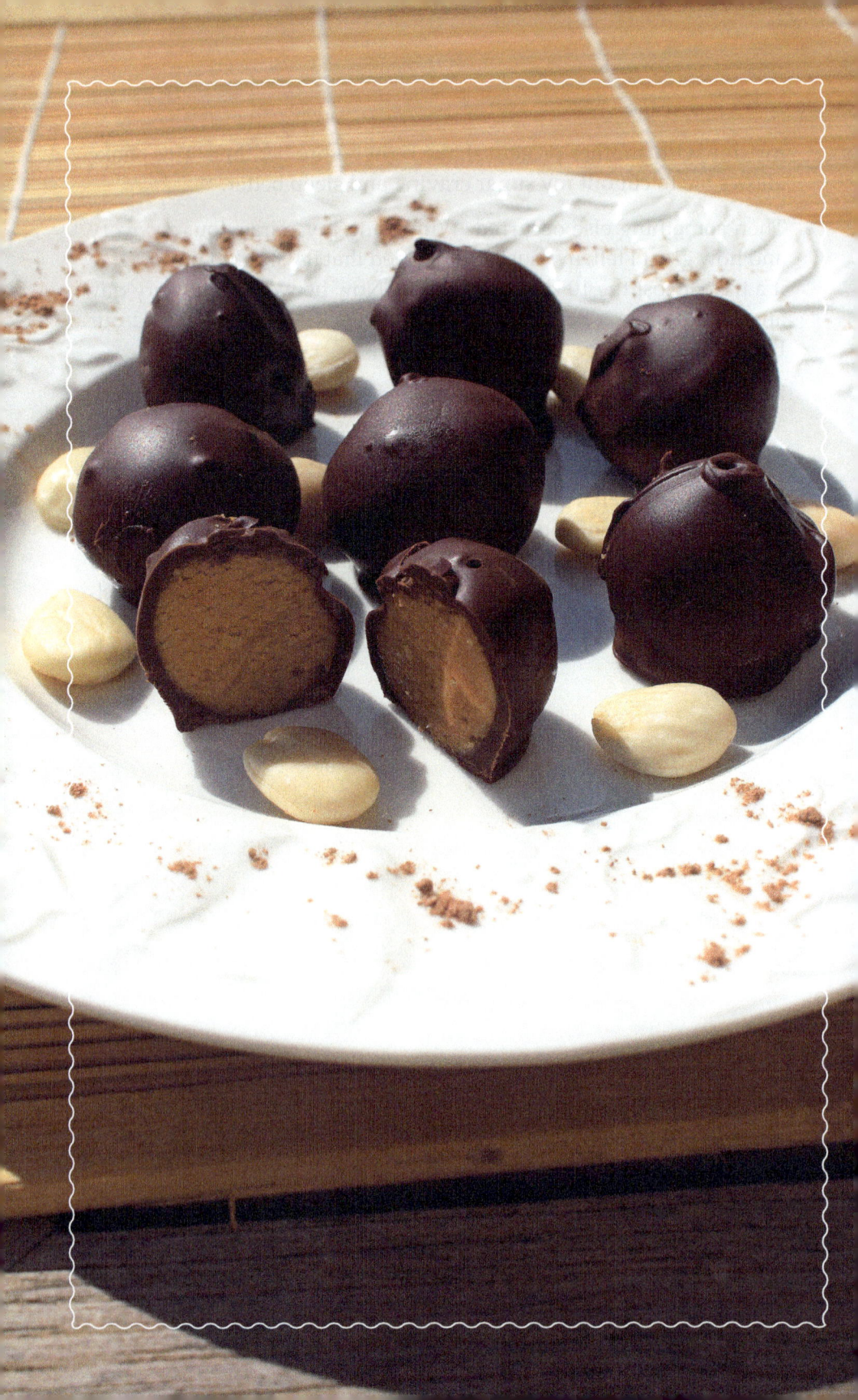

CHOCOLATE HEAVEN BALLS

Ingredients:

- 1 cup bio peanut butter
- 1/2 cup of raw almond flour
- 1 spoon Maca powder
- 1/2 spoon ginger powder
- 1 spoon Agave syrup
- 2 cups of bio chocolate (73 percent)

Directions:

Mix all the ingredients with a fork. Store in the refrigerator for 15 minutes until the mixture is firmer. Then start forming 1-inch balls and place them on a cookie sheet. Freeze for one hour. Meanwhile, warm the chocolate in a "bain-marie" until melted. Remove balls from freezer, and using a toothpick, delicately dip each one into the melted chocolate and replace back onto the cookie sheet. Place them back into the refrigerator so the chocolate becomes firm again.

Enjoy!

ZUCCHINI AND BROCCOLI POTAGE

Ingredients:

- 3 zucchini
- 1 broccoli head
- 1 cup raw white almonds
- Parsley
- Himalayan salt and pepper to taste
- Bio soya cream

Directions:

First, let the raw white almonds soak in water for 2 hours. This will clean them and especially make them a bit tender. Then reduce them to a flour-like substance using a food processor. Clean, peel, and cut the zucchini, clean and cut the broccoli, and place everything in a pot until cooked. They should still be a bit firm. Drain the water and place them into a soup bowl. Add the salt and pepper, the almonds, and mix it all until smooth. Lastly, add the parsley and mix slightly again.

Serve in bowls with a bit of bio soya cream. It's delicious.

COMPILED BY **HEATHER EDEN**

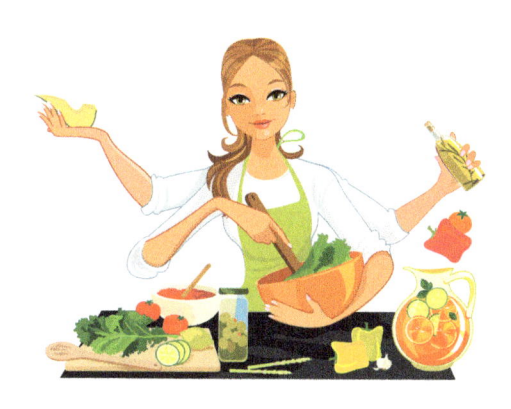

Fawn MacMichael, CHHC, AADP

Fawn MacMichael is a certified holistic health and wellness coach, certified through the Institute for Integrative Nutrition, and accredited through the American Association of Drugless Practitioners. She is also working toward a raw food chef certification. Fawn uses her own health journey of healing, knowledge, and research, along with her training in various dietary methods and theories to guide her clients on their own journey to health. Fawn's passion for "healthifying" recipes to meet her family's dietary needs, and detoxifying the home, the kitchen, and life also empowers her clients to make lasting lifestyle changes.

- www.fawnmacmichael.com
- www.facebook.com/pages/Naturally-Empowered-with-Fawn-MacMichael/
- www.pinterest.com/healthymomma18/
- naturallyempowered@gmail.com

PRACTICE 10

Sacred Source Eating (Organic, Clean, Real)

By Fawn MacMichael, CHHC, AADP

Think back to our ancestors many generations ago. They ate real food—food that was free of all toxic fertilizers, pesticides, fungicides, chemicals, additives, artificial ingredients, and chemical preservatives. The diseases and ailments that are so common now were not common back then. We really need to get back to this way of life. Backyard gardens are one way to do this. There is such satisfaction in being barefoot in nature, touching the Earth's soil and feeling it's energy, harvesting the produce and eating it. Our food has energy. Think about a plant when it grows—it capture's energy from the sun. That's why it's so important to eat foods close to harvest time, so we get the most energy from it.

I have learned that we truly are what we eat, absorb, and are exposed to. Our bodies can't do what they are supposed to and function properly if they aren't being fed what God has made for us. When fed quality, organic foods, our bodies can thrive, heal themselves of many ailments/diseases, and be filled with life and energy. I was the average American, consuming what many people would consider normal. If it was convenient, tasted decent, and the package seemed to portray a healthier choice, I ate it. But a time came when I was sick and tired of feeling sick and tired. So I decided to seek truth in what is actually in our food, where is comes from, what is added to it, and how all of this affects the body.

If you rewind a few years prior, I was depressed, sick often, on prescriptions and non-prescriptions (some for years and multiple short-term), had many doctor appointments, was exhausted (drinking a pot of coffee a day!), and had a host of daily ailments. I thought this was normal. Up until then, I never thought about food or how the quality of food affects our bodies, both positively or negatively, depending on the choices we make.

Along my journey to health (that I am currently still on), I realized that a lot of my life had been a combination of poor eating and lifestyle choices, as well as childhood exposure to a variety of insecticides that damaged my body. It was at that point, I realized just how important organic clean living is. Eating the way God intended affects so many aspects of how the body functions. Our bodies were created perfectly by God. And he has provided the perfect nutrients to nourish and help heal our bodies. Realizing this was such an "a-ha" moment for me.

Not long after switching to organic, my family started to get rid of most ailments and symptoms. Slowly, we stopped needing prescriptions or doctor appointments, and we weren't sick and tired anymore. Note: My family and I eat organic, but we also eat what we feel is "clean." We've taken out foods, products, and chemicals that are toxic and/or inflammatory to the body. Instead, we choose organic produce, nuts and seeds, herbs, spices, quality grass-fed meats, naturally sweet foods for added sweetness, superfoods for added vitality, and natural household and body care products. Once switching to this way of eating and living, we haven't looked back.

Kids adapt very well, but it takes time to allow their taste buds to adjust. Including them in the kitchen and allowing them to be part of the process really connects them to the food. Allowing them to see you make quality food a priority, and being open with them about the truth, has a huge impact. They learn about true health, healing, and that God has provided all of this for us. My family also balances this with our spiritual beliefs and prayer. We believe we do what we can, and know that Jesus can do what we can't. He heals above and beyond what we are able to.

After learning of the toxic childhood exposures, I also realized it was detrimental to my health and healing to eat 100 percent organic and reduce toxic exposures of all kinds. Conventional foods specifically have toxic chemicals that cause bodily malfunctions. They disrupt our endocrine system, hormones, organs, bodily functions, system communications, cause negative cell and gene expressions, and can cause cancer as well as diseases. This affects us and generations after us. Also, by choosing organic, it supports organic farmers, sustainable agriculture, avoids exposure to toxic chemicals and GMO's, it's safer for the environment, and it saves animals, insects (bees especially), and aquatic life.

Did you know there are hidden toxins in conventional foods? Conventional meat and dairy have hormones, antibiotics, GMO's, bacteria, bleach, ammonia, and more. Conventional produce is sprayed with chemicals and the soil it's grown in is lacking most minerals needed for the produce to be full of vitamins and minerals. Packaged foods in the stores are filled with these conventional foods for a portion of the ingredients, but also have preservatives, additives, poor quality fillers, "enriched" ingredients, addictive substances (MSG, sugar, etc.), and artificial colors/flavors/sweeteners. All of these are toxic, and the food labels often trick us. Our bodies don't recognize these ingredients, and when trying to process them, it actually depletes our bodies of vitamins and minerals.

We are all exposed to toxins daily that our body has to try to filter out or store in our cells (fat cells, fatty tissue glands, and organs). From carpet, furniture, and draperies to cellular radiation and pollution, we are all exposed every day. We live in a less than perfect world. But I believe that if we do what we can, by nourishing our bodies with the foods, herbs, spices, oils, and superfoods that the Lord has provided for us, it will support our bodies to better handle the daily worldly toxins. Adding plants to the home to help filter toxins, using nontoxic home and body care products, drinking quality water, and addressing lifestyle factors can all add up to better overall health. With better overall health, the body can more easily deal with and eliminate toxins we are exposed to.

Eating clean, organic real food will nourish and feed every cell of the body, giving us optimal health. It allows not only healing and nourishment, but it lifts the toxic fog. This allows the brain to think clearer. We start to really see, think, and feel differently. It really is a sacred way of eating, by connecting the body, mind, and soul.

These recipes I'm sharing use quality ingredients that support health and nourish the body.

TROPICAL CHOCOLATE PORRIDGE PUDDING

Serves 4 to 5

Ingredients:

- 2 1/2 to 3 cups almond or coconut milk
- 1 tsp. alcohol-free vanilla extract (or other flavor)
- 1 tsp. cinnamon
- 1/2 cup chia seeds
- 1/3 cup unsweetened shredded coconut
- 4 tbsp. nut butter of choice (or a mixture)
- 1/8 cup plus 1/16 cup Raw Cacao
- 2 tbsp. hemp seeds
- 1 tbsp. quality unflavored gelatin (I recommend Great Lakes brand, the pink/reddish orange can—not the green can, it won't "gel.")
- 4 tbsp. local honey or maple syrup

*Or, for a sugar-free option, 2 droppers of liquid stevia (or to taste)

Add-ins of choice: Goji berries, chopped nuts, pumpkin, fruit, spices, etc.

Directions:

Place all ingredients into a small pot on the stove, over med-low heat. Stir until mixed together, approximately 2 to 4 minutes. Serve immediately. Store leftovers in the fridge. Optionally, you could mix ingredients in a bowl, without heating, and then place in the fridge to chill before serving. This recipe is very versatile. If it's too thick, add more liquid. If it's too runny, add more chia seeds or gelatin.

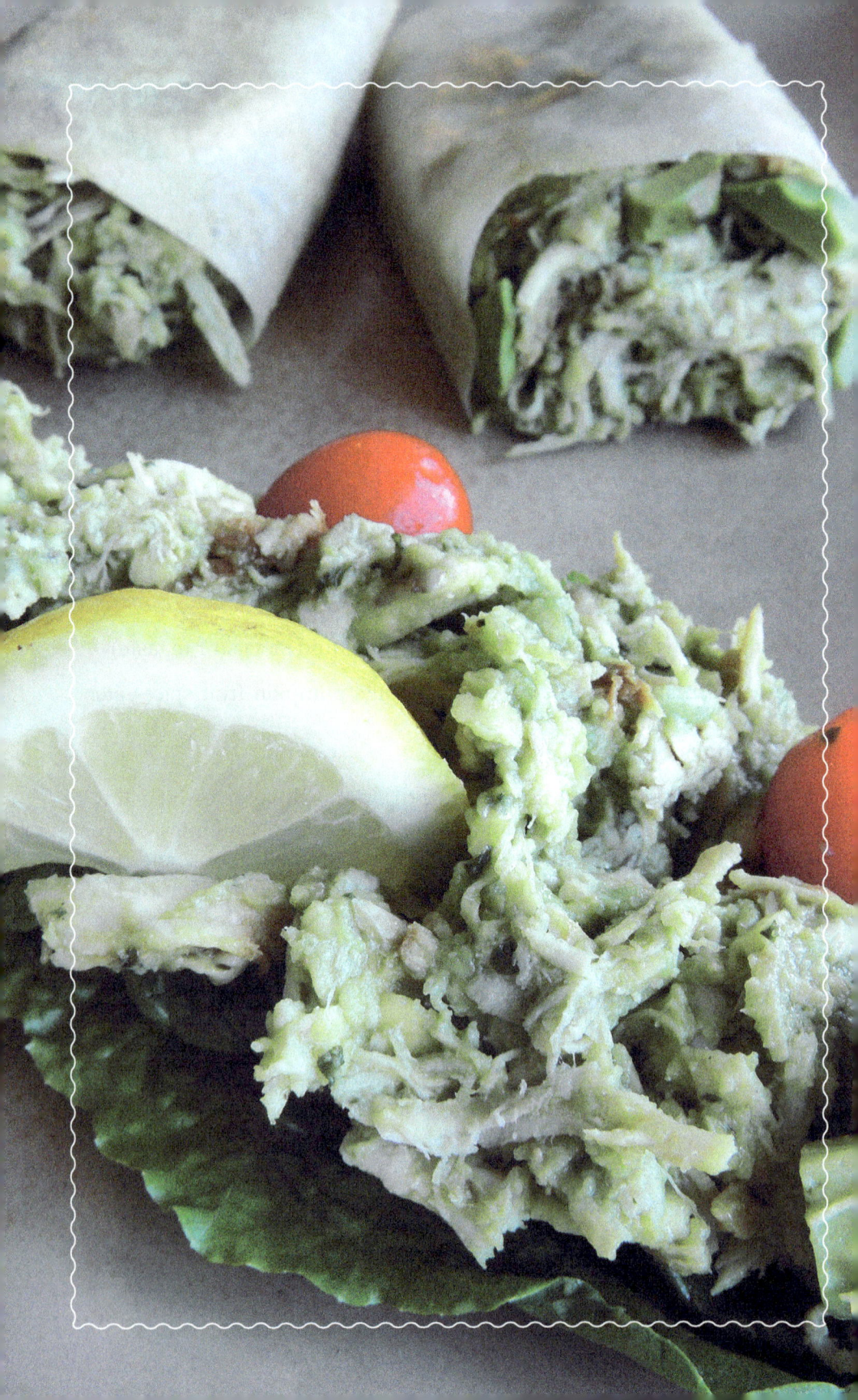

TROPICAL AVO-CHICKEN SALAD WRAPS

Serves 4 to 5

Ingredients:

- 1 lb. chicken
- 10 shakes coconut aminos
- 2 ripe avocados
- 1/8 tsp. garlic powder (plus a few dashes)
- 1/8 tsp. onion powder (plus a few dashes)
- Pepper and Himalayan salt to taste
- Juice of 1 lime or lemon
- 1 tbsp. dried cilantro
- Julian Bakery "Paleo (coconut) wraps" (available in select health food stores and on Amazon)
- Lettuce or leafy green of choice
- Sprouts and veggies of choice

Directions:

Cook chicken in a skillet over medium heat, with coconut aminos and a few dashes of garlic and onion powders. Cover and let cook about 5 to 8 minutes. Flip the chicken, cover, and let cook another 5 to 8 minutes or until cooked through. Let the chicken cool and then shred into a bowl. While the chicken is cooking and cooling, you can make the avocado mixture. In a bowl, mash the avocados. Add the seasonings, cilantro, and citrus juice. Taste and add more seasonings as needed. Scoop the avocado mixture into the shredded chicken. Stir to thoroughly combine. You can serve this chicken salad over lettuce or in a wrap. If using the Paleo coconut wraps, scoop the chicken salad into the wrap. Add veggies, and/or sprouts of choice. Roll the wrap and enjoy! Or you can simply scoop the chicken salad over lettuce and add the veggies and/or sprouts you'd like. Serve with soup or roasted sweet potato bites.

COMPILED BY **HEATHER EDEN**

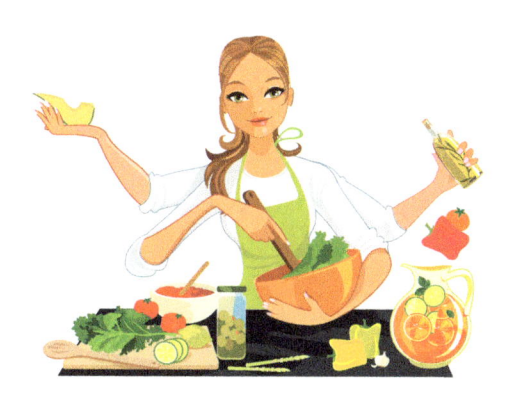

Tosca Page

Tosca Page is a health enthusiast! She loves empowering others and giving them healthy alternative solutions. It can be so hard to live a healthy lifestyle if you're surrounded by unhealthy people. And it takes an incredible amount of courage to try alternative things—like natural birth, home remedies, etc.—when well-meaning people are telling you that something bad is going to happen to you and your children if you don't follow their advice. Tosca Page is here to provide simple healthy solutions that make living a healthy lifestyle easy for the whole family.

- www.RawHealthNut.com
- tosca@rawhealthnut.com
- www.facebook.com/LittleHealthNut
- www.twitter.com/ToscaPage
- Tosca Page

PRACTICE 11

Healthy Proteins

By Tosca Page

When my oldest son first started eating solids, like most moms, I wanted to make sure that he got all the nutrients that he needed. The big one that everyone talks about is protein! I was leaning towards a vegan diet for our family, but I was concerned about my son getting enough protein. So, I poured over books and picked every health conscious person's brain that I could find. Finally, the pieces of the puzzle started coming together, and my first "a-ha!" moment came when I realized that all raw fruits and vegetables have a certain amount of protein in them. After lots of research, I started to see that we shouldn't be focused on trying to get isolated nutrients, like more protein, vitamin C, etc.—if we eat a variety of healthy foods, we will get all of these nutrients in the perfect balance for our bodies to easily assimilate and utilize anyway. And once I learned about the immense nutritional content of superfoods, my worries about protein were completely gone. When we eat lots of fresh, organic produce, nuts, seeds, and superfoods, our body has everything that it needs to do well! Here are some of the wonderful sources of protein that I have found:

SUPERFOODS

Hemp seeds: There are 10 grams of protein in just 4 tbsp of raw, organic hemp seeds. They also contain all ten essential amino acids, making them a complete protein. They offer a perfect balance of Omega 3, 6, and 9 and are a great source of magnesium, iron, and zinc.

Spirulina: This amazing freshwater algae is the highest form of protein found anywhere in the world! It's even higher than some fish and beef

(up to 73 percent! salmon is a close second at 62 percent and beef has 37 percent.)

To better understand this, here are the calculations of proteins as a percentage of calories—when you're doing a calorie breakdown, the protein, fat, and carb ratios all add up to 100 percent. This gives you a better understanding of what percentage of protein your food is actually made of:

- Salmon: 38 percent fat, 0 percent carbs, **62 percent protein**
- translate to serving size: 1 cup – 166 calories, 6.72g fat, 0g carbs, 24.52g protein
- Beef: 63 percent fat, 0 percent carbs, **37 percent protein**
- translate to serving size: 1 cup – 348 calories, 23.64g fat, 0g carbs, 31.86g protein
- Spirulina: 0 percent fat, 27 percent carbs, **73 percent protein**
- translate to serving size: 1 tbsp. – 25 calories, 0g fat, 1.5g carbs, 4g protein

Spirulina protein is up to 95 percent digestible, (meaning that your body can utilize it), making it one of the highest digestible vegetarian proteins out there.

Other protein-rich superfoods: Chlorella 58.4 percent, dulse 50 percent, bee pollen 31 percent, Goji berries 18 percent, Maca powder 20 percent, chia seeds 15 percent, and kelp 10 percent.

NUTS AND SEEDS

Pumpkin seeds: One ounce of pumpkin seeds contains 9.35 grams of protein! That's over two grams more than the same quantity of ground beef. They are also full of vitamin K, vitamin E, folate, calcium, iron, zinc, and more.

Almonds: There are 20 grams of protein in 1 cup of almonds. They are also an excellent source of vitamin E, iron, potassium, and calcium.

Other protein-rich nuts and seeds: (Serving size 1 cup): sesame seeds 25g, sunflower seeds 29g, flax seeds 26g, walnuts 15g, Brazil nuts 19g, and pine nuts 18g.

VEGETABLES, SPROUTS, AND BEANS

Even vegetables have protein in them!

Green peas: Contain 20 percent protein (7.86g per cup! That's about the same as a cup of milk). They are also rich in vitamin K, B1, folic acid, and antioxidants.

Alfalfa sprouts: Contain 35 percent protein (1.9g per cup) and are an abundant source of vitamins A, B, C, E and K, calcium, chlorophyll, amino acids, and trace elements.

Other protein-rich veggies and sprouts: Red clover sprouts 42 percent, broccoli sprouts 35 percent, cauliflower 21 percent, and collard greens 18 percent.

Mung bean: Has 14 grams of protein in just 1 cup and are a rich source of fiber, vitamin C, potassium, zinc, and folic acid.

Other beans: (Service size 1 cup): Lentils 18g, navy beans 15g, kidney beans 13g, garbanzo beans 15g, and pinto beans 11g.

There are so many protein sources out there that are packed with incredible nutrients, designed to give our bodies everything we need. I recommend you buy these protein sources raw and organic! When food is cooked or processed, essential nutrients like vitamins, minerals, and enzymes are lost. Amino acids—the building blocks of protein—begin to deteriorate and are completely destroyed at 160 degrees.

QUICK MORNING BREAKFAST SMOOTHIE

I love green smoothies! They are a perfect on-the-go meal and you can make them in less than five minutes. Here is one of our family favorites:

Serving size: 5 cups

Ingredients:

- 2 cups of raw greens (kale or spinach works best)
- 3 bananas (frozen is better)
- 4 cups of apple juice (cold is best)
- 1 tbsp. superfood of your choice (chia seeds, hemp seeds, spirulina, etc.)
- 1 cup of ice (2 cups if your fruit isn't frozen)
- 2 1/2 cups of frozen berries (I love Trader Joes Organic Mixed Berry Blend—with strawberries, blackberries, raspberries, and blueberries.)

Directions:

Blend on high until smooth and creamy. Serve with a straw and enjoy!

Tips:

Get yourself a good superfood! Hemp seeds and chia seeds are a great way to start your day, because they are loaded with nutrients that will give you sustained energy and will leave you feeling satisfied.

Buy your ingredients raw and organic! Organic has up to 300 percent more vitamins and minerals than conventionally grown foods, so you won't need to use as much. The superfoods may be a little more expensive, but they should last you a long time. The reason that it's important to buy your superfoods raw is because there are so many amazing phytonutrients, vitamins, minerals, and immune-boosting properties that get destroyed or damaged when processed.

Use cold ingredients! This can make the difference between a good or bad tasting smoothie. One thing I do is buy lots of bananas, peel them, and throw them in the freezer, and this makes my smoothies extra cold and sweet.

I hope you enjoy this delicious smoothie as much as our family does. It's a great way to sneak nutrition into your day!

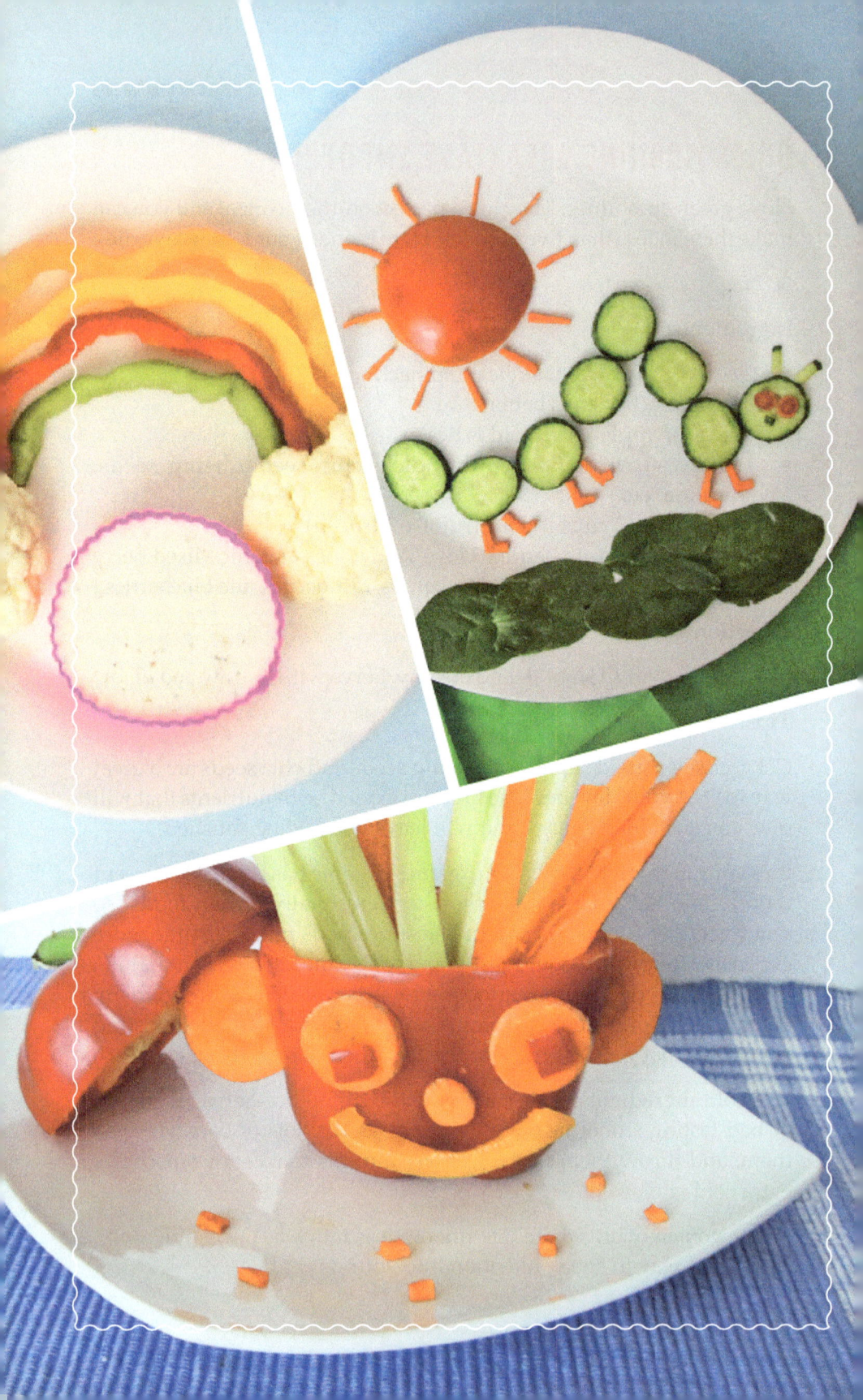

COMPILED BY **HEATHER EDEN**

VEGGIE ART

One of my secrets to getting my children to want to eat their veggies is to make it fun! Your children may not eat what you make the first, second, or even tenth time, but that's totally fine! Just keep it fun, and you will see they'll start to have a great relationship with healthy food.

Here are some tips:

- At first, pick veggies that they like and then you can slowly introduce new veggies.

- You can make this a creative activity that you and your children do together, or it can be a fun, quick snack.

- If they don't eat anything, don't sweat it! You can always use the veggies for something else later. The key is to create a positive environment where they don't feel pressured.

- Make a big deal about the things they create! Show it to family, take a picture, etc.

- Give them their veggie snack when they're hungry—a great time is when lunch or dinner is cooking, especially after they've just finished doing a physical activity.

- I always keep veggies and the main course separate! That way I don't need to battle to get them to eat their veggies. When there are cooked foods and sauces on the plate, raw veggies can seem bland.

- Create a daily routine that's conducive to eating healthy. If you're always running around and grabbing unhealthy options, then it's going to be hard for your children to reach for the healthy stuff. You will have a lot more success by planning your day in a way that makes time for healthy snacks. For example, healthy veggie snacks are always around 10:30 a.m. for us. I start cooking lunch and prepare them a fun snack to munch on while I'm cooking. You'll be surprised it doesn't actually take that long to throw something together that looks fun, once you get into the habit of it. If we're at the playground, I chop up some raw veggies beforehand and put them in snack sized Ziploc bags. They are always hungry after they're done playing, so it makes a great snack on the ride home, before lunchtime.

I hope these tips help! If you can create a fun, positive environment around healthy foods, they will gravitate towards them time and time again. It may take time to get into the groove of things, but don't give up! Eating healthy is a lifestyle and takes time. You may think all the work you put in isn't working, but it is. You've planted the seed, now watch it grow!

COMPILED BY **HEATHER EDEN**

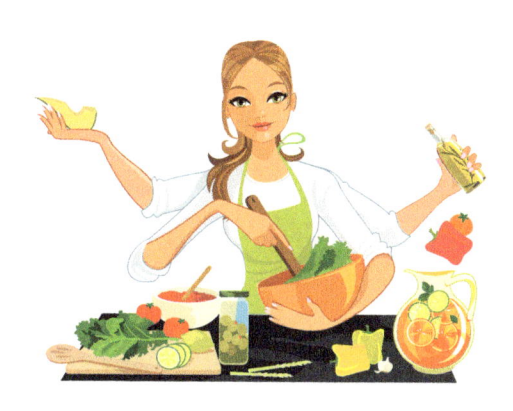

Rachel Miller, CHHC, AADP, CPT, PTA

Rachel Miller is a certified holistic health coach, certified personal trainer, and certified Pilates instructor. After transforming her life by losing over one hundred pounds and keeping it off for thirteen years, she hopes to use her experience to make an impact on her clients and help them feel as great as she does. Her fitness and nutrition success stories have been featured on a local news station in Buffalo, NY. She is the founder of Reform with Rachel, where she focuses on weight loss issues and designs individualized nutrition and fitness programs for her clients.

- 716.380.0738
- fitness201@verizon.net
- www.reformwithrachel.com
- www.facebook.com/ReformWithRachel

PRACTICE 12

Eating With Self-Respect

By Rachel Miller, CHHC, AAD, CPT, PTA

My memories of being overweight go back to the eighth grade. I always felt self- conscious. People would make comments behind my back. Family and friends would even confront me about my weight. I didn't date like all my friends. I struggled inside, but never let it show—always portraying happiness.

I reached my heaviest weight in college. I realized being overweight as an adult was not any easier than it was as a teen. However, it was concerning to me, and something had to be done. I began experimenting with different diets, such as Atkins and Weight Watchers. When each fad was over, I learned that diets didn't work long-term. So I did things my way. I started cutting down my portions and eliminating diet soda. I started taking long walks, which eventually turned into running five miles a day. I also incorporated workout videos at home. I didn't belong to a gym, never used diet pills, or ever had any surgeries to lose weight. I made exercise a priority and stopped finding excuses.

The weight started to come off little by little. I was feeling great physically, mentally, and for the first time, emotionally! After two years, I had lost one hundred pounds. I am proud to have kept off the weight, plus more, for over thirteen years. I am proud of who I have become.

Finding balance between eating for nourishment, eating for enjoyment, and eating for emotional reasons has been the key to my success. This is my formula:

WHAT TO EAT

This could be as simple as learning what kinds of foods are right for your individual body. Everybody is unique and requires different things. The foods I used to eat, such as fast and processed foods, would deplete my energy, suppress my immune system, and often reflect negative emotions.

Over time, I have learned to choose healthier foods like vegetables, lean protein, beans, fish, and a lot of water. These provide nourishment, help me sleep better, and give me the energy my body requires. I also exercise on a regular basis.

When we think of food in terms of numbers or points, we forget to take into account the nutrients, the taste, and the reason we are consuming it in the first place. We forget to enjoy it.

LISTEN TO YOUR BODY AND FOLLOW YOUR INSTINCTS

Now I eat when I am truly hungry, not because it's lunchtime or because I want dessert, even though I am already full. We can learn from how a baby eats. They cry when they are hungry and stop when they have had enough.

Some days you may feel hungry more frequently, and rarely the next. This is your body's way of telling you to adjust your caloric intake accordingly.

I like the saying, "If you eat when you are not hungry, how will you know when to stop?"

ACKNOWLEDGE *WHY* YOU ARE EATING

We eat for many reasons, including social gatherings and special occasions. We also tend to eat when we are bored, tired, depressed, stressed, or even happy. Our emotions then take over our eating habits and patterns. Are you eating to suppress feelings of a broken marriage, a death, or unhappy career?

I have become more aware of my actions and feelings around food. I ask myself *why* I am about to grab that snack. I find that it is because I am stressed or bored. Asking myself "Am I hungry?" has really helped me control my emotional eating instead of turning to food for comfort. I also ask myself how I want to feel afterward.

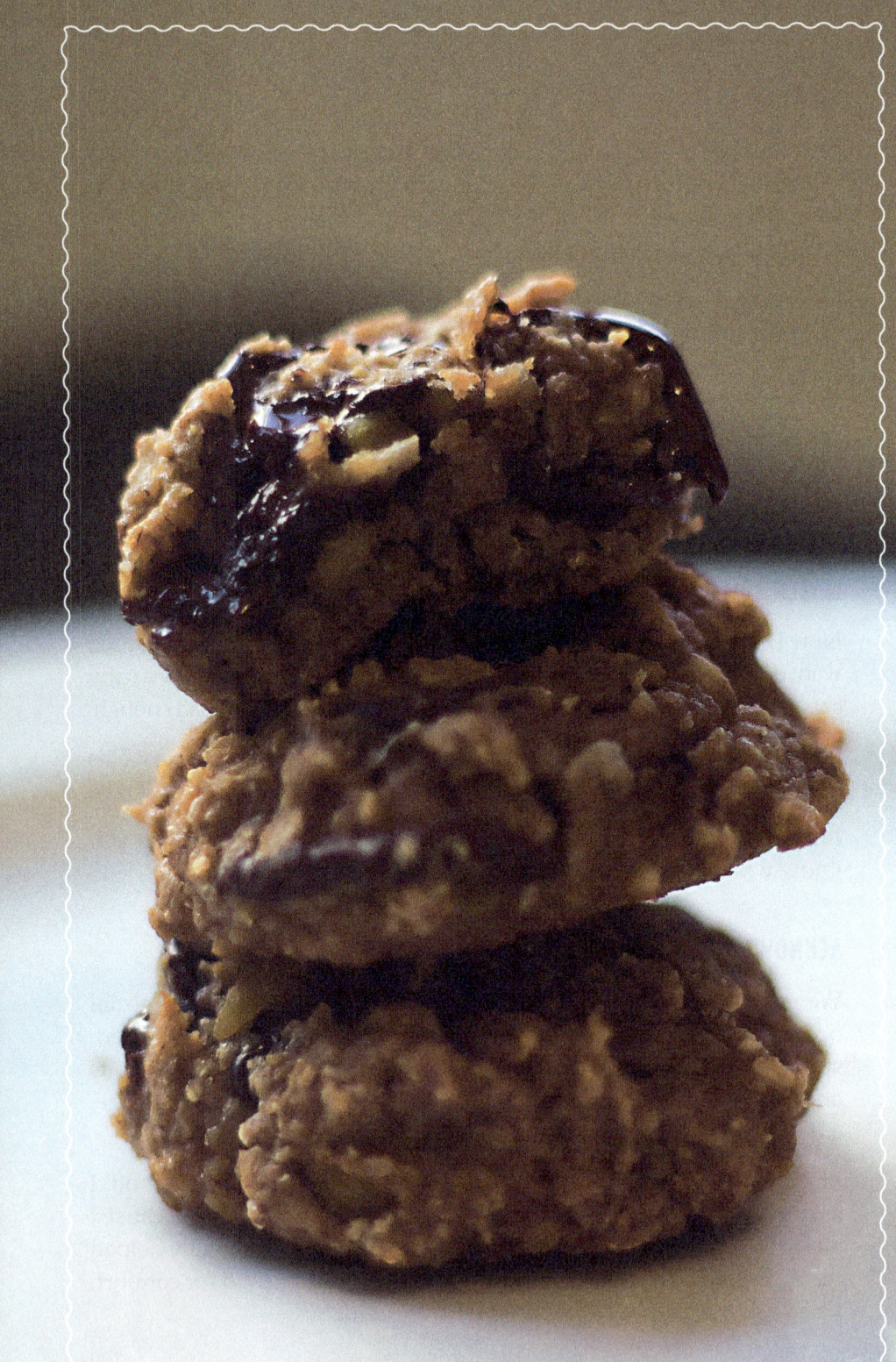

STRIVE FOR OPTIMAL HEALTH

Most people think of being healthy as physical—consisting of nutrition and exercise. But to me it also involves spirituality. This is finding the ability to love the person you are right now, whether you are a size 2 or 22. It is dealing with the real, deep down issues at hand. I am learning how to develop a positive relationship with myself and not covering it up with food.

Going through this process has inspired me to make a career out of health and wellness. I became a certified holistic health coach, and I also hold certifications in STOTT Pilates, as well as personal training. Juggling two children, instructing fitness and Pilates classes, and running my own health coaching business, I am always looking for quick healthy meals for my family.

The nutrients in foods we choose for our families support our day-to-day living. They will affect how you feel now and in the future. Not having enough nutrients will lead to developing diseases and additional health problems.

Get your children involved with preparing meals, eat together as much as possible, and offer a variety of snacks. I encourage and educate my children on healthy eating habits so they will become happy and confident adults, and have a healthy relationship with food. Here are some goals to strive for:

PREPARE FOODS THAT GIVE YOUR FAMILY ENERGY

Make meals and snacks that nourish you and your children all day long. Indulging in too many snacks, processed foods, and drive-thrus will cause fatigue, moodiness, and suppress the immune system.

NOTICE HOW YOUR FAMILY EATS

Are they eating because they are bored? It is important to sit down as a family and enjoy the meal you have prepared.

Practicing techniques on what, when, why, and how you eat will have the whole family feeling better physically, mentally, and emotionally.

COMPILED BY **HEATHER EDEN**

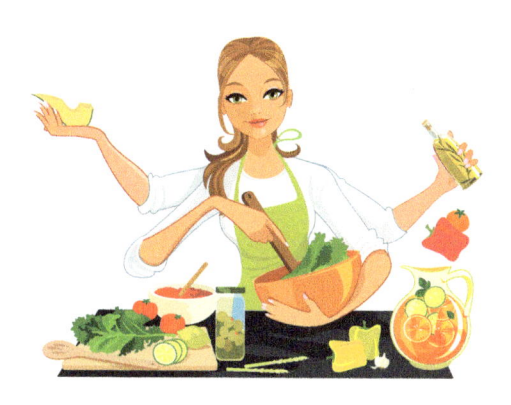

Sarah Mastriani-Levi, CHHC, AADP, RYT

Sarah Mastriani-Levi, creator of Mannafest Living, serves as an international holistic health coach and personal chef. She is often referred to as a boldly authentic spiritual pioneer, creative visionary and inspirational catalyst. She lectures internationally and offers workshops and holistic health coaching for the health-curious to the avidly health-conscious.

Parallel to her holistic consulting and various food services, she actively homeschools her four children as a single parent, raising them with a strong bond to nature. She has raised them in an ecological manner, in harmony with nature. Her children have grown from all of the fresh goodness that nature has to offer, both physically and spiritually.

- www.mannafest-living.com
- contact@mannafest-living.com
- www.facebook.com/organic.veggie.girl
- www.facebook.com/MannafestLiving
- Sarah Mastriani-Levi, Personal Chef and Holistic Health Coach

PRACTICE 13

The Sacred Kitchen

By Sarah Mastriani-Levi, CHHC, AADP, RYT

What is feeding your soul? What are you hungry for?

Love? Gratitude? Acknowledgement? Validation? Expression?

All of these things can be found through experience in our kitchens and souls.

How we "do" food is how we "do" everything. So for all of you who either "don't like the kitchen" or "don't have the time to invest in food prep," I want to encourage you to take a look within yourself and really ask, "Why?"

Have you convinced yourself it is too difficult or complicated? Do you enjoy the food but loathe the cleanup? Could the real answer be that you don't know how to prepare things so everything is a new learning project? Perhaps you come home tired from a long day and just want a quick fix to stop the cries coming from hungry bellies. Maybe you know you could do more but just can't seem to wrap your brain around the time-management issue. Are you riddled with guilty feelings of insufficiency?

These are all things I hear from clients on a daily basis, with the most common sentence being, "Well, I try to eat healthy." Everyone absolutely feels they're doing the best they can. Trying is not enough, because it lacks true awareness.

MAKING ARTISTRY OF OUR OWN EXISTENCE

We each have received a unique opportunity in our lifetime to make a difference and to initiate change in our surroundings. We are each given a different skill set. It is our obligation to give back to the Universe by using the skills and talents that are naturally available to us.

Yet we all require one thing in common to make change...fuel.

What kind of fuel seems to be the real question? In order to find the answer to this and other tricky questions, we must first look within. Often, we don't want to deal with emotions hidden beneath bad eating habits like bingeing, purging, dieting, and ingesting processed comfort foods. Emotional eating is one of the leading causes of nutritional imbalances in the Western world. However, without facing these hidden issues, we are doomed to repeat them endlessly until ill health puts a stop to it.

I have found it is very difficult to have a spiritual shift in perception without having a physical shift in perception. Here's an exercise that serves as a catalyst for cleaning out the areas we don't want and allows ourselves access within our own consciousness and assists in facing how we view the world.

FACING THE REALITY OF WHAT'S HIDDEN AWAY

I visit clients' homes for "kitchen interventions" and take everything out of their pantries and cabinets. We put it all on the floor in front of them. They are then asked to divide their food into three categories: one they consider healthy food, one they consider non-healthy food, and one of allowable snacks. This process forces them to see what they're hoarding and supplying for emotional eating binges, comfort foods, quick snacks, and what they believe is nutritional. This is a fantastic exercise not only for taking stock of what you have in your cabinets, but also for taking stock of what you don't want to see about yourself that's hiding in your closet. We then move on from there into the refrigerator and freezer and any other places they might have "food stashes" hiding. If things aren't flowing in the kitchen, there's a reason. Either they're doing it just like their moms or grandmas did, without giving it much thought, or they have so much clutter they just don't have any idea how to pull things together to make a meal.

I highly recommend simplifying in every way possible. Food should have a constant turnover, both in your refrigerator and in your pantry. Stop holding onto old food and dishes that create clutter—they stop the flow of new energy into your space. Instead, invest your time, money, and tendency to keep things with a garden. Understand that a garden has transient timelessness that connects you to the sacred. Each time you pick fruits, vegetables, and herbs to eat from your garden, fresh energy feeds your soul. When you don't take time to feed your soul with the proper nourishment, what you get is a processed lifestyle and a huge disconnect from the divine. Freshness will inspire you and turn on your creativity. It will connect you to the sacred.

ORGANIZING YOUR WORK SPACE

My kitchen is my workshop, my temple…where I create my artistry. I practice the art form of soul nourishment. It's where I come to worship and how I connect to the divine. For many of you, that probably sounds like "woo woo." After all, when you come home from work all you want to do is to get something to eat and take a break from everything you've done all day.

You too can connect to the sacred and communicate with the divine by:

- Slowing down, meditating, and observing nature.
- Feeding your soul with the freshness that has the primary energy still existing in plants. Fruits, vegetables, raw nuts, and seeds are all full of divine energy. They calm your spirit, relax your body, and return you to your natural element.
- Going outside to find a place where it's quiet.
- Breathing fresh air.
- Leaving your media at home, allowing your breath, the wind, and the leaves to be your music.
- Lighting a candle in your kitchen to bring in the divine pure fire element to create connection.

CREATING GRATITUDE AND AWARENESS

Begin each food prep session with gratitude. Allow your body to guide you as you start to become aware of what feels good. Take note of what foods make you feel fantastic. When you bring your awareness to your food, suddenly the awareness expands into other parts of your life and enables you to bring joy to what you love. Awareness will begin to proliferate into the rest of your life, by respecting how it feels in your body. You will suddenly *know* what you are feeling.

Stop living and eating like you need to prepare for the end of the world, and start living like you want to feed your soul with authentic awareness for the rest of your life.

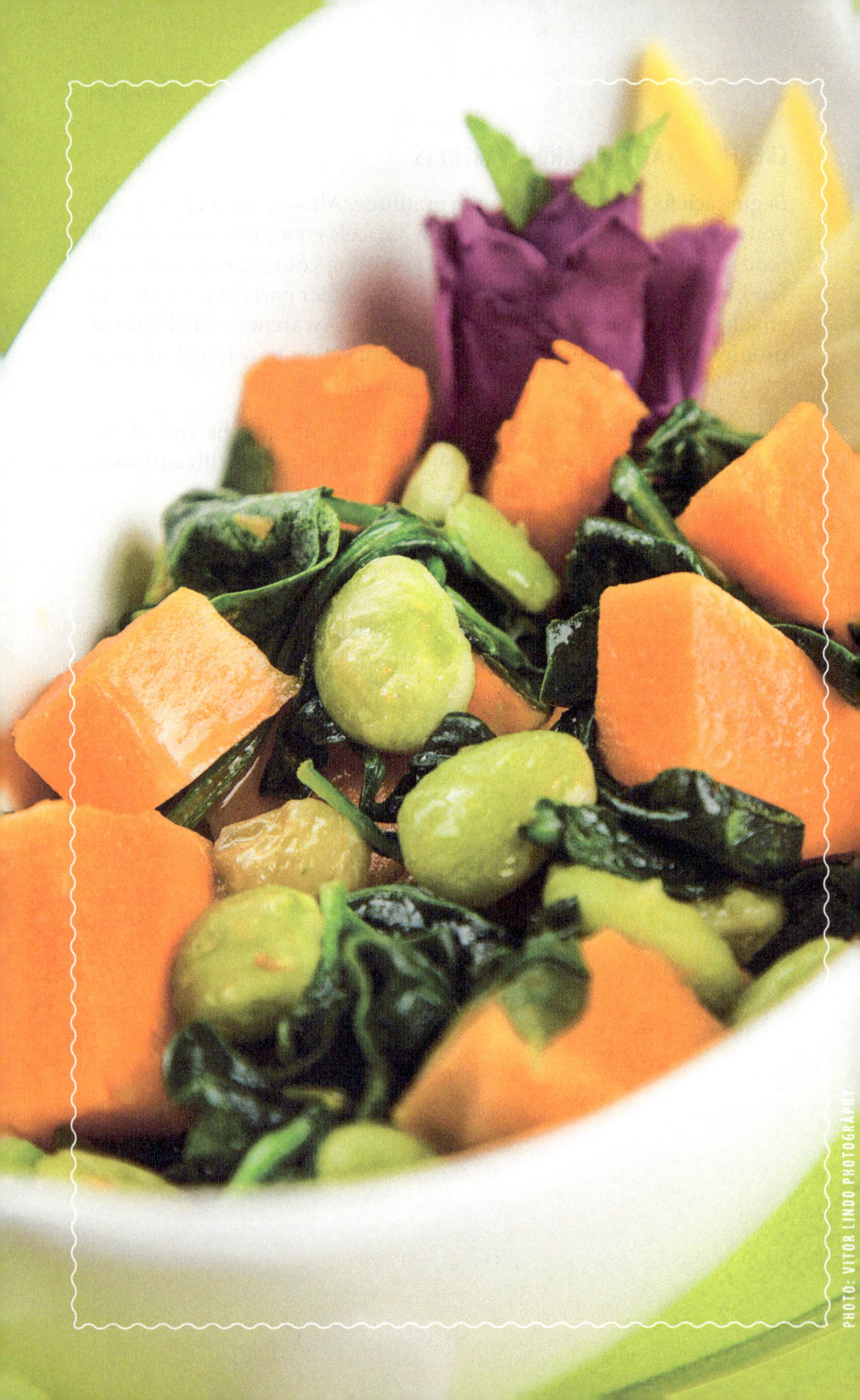

BUTTERNUT SQUASH WITH LIMA BEANS AND BABY SPINACH

Butternut squash is packed with anti-inflammatory nutrients, rich in Omega 3's and beta-carotene, which keep the immune system in top form to offer protection from colds and flu. They are super easy to grow. Lima beans, also known as butterbeans, are great for stabilizing blood sugar levels and providing a steady source of energy. Baby spinach is chock-full of vital energy, vitamin C, and alkalizing green goodness. Be careful to maintain the ultra-bright green color achieved by the super quick cooking time, by adding it last to this recipe and not leaving it covered after the 1 1/2 minutes. Pure goodness in a super quick meal.

Ingredients:

- 1 large organic butternut squash (peeled and cut into 3/4 inch cubes)
- 4 cups of cooked lima beans (firm, yet tender) or 1 bag of frozen lima beans
- 18 to 24 oz. of fresh organic baby spinach
- 1 tbsp. of sea salt
- 1/2 tsp. ground coriander
- 2 to 3 cloves of garlic (minced)
- 2 to 3 tbsp. of cold-pressed extra virgin olive oil

Directions:

In a large wok, add olive oil and minced garlic. Immediately, add the butternut squash cubes and thoroughly combine with the garlic and olive oil. Sauté for 3 to 5 minutes over medium-high heat. Add the lima beans. Incorporate into the mixture and cover for 2 minutes. Add the baby spinach and cover for 1 1/2 minutes. Remove from the heat source and uncover. Add the sea salt and ground coriander. Enjoy immediately while bright green. Offer thanks.

SIMPLE GARDEN PESTO

I venture into the garden to pick a few sprigs of basil, cilantro, parsley, mint, and some garlic chives. I bring them into the house, rinse and place them on a cutting board. I add a handful of pumpkin seeds and some sea salt and start with my knife, working a back-and-forth *chop-chop-chop* until it becomes nice and smooth. I gather it all into a bowl and add some olive oil for an instant pesto. I serve it with some Ezekiel bread and cucumber slices. Instantly, the energy of the garden's freshness is available to be eaten. I light a candle and give thanks and gratitude. By mindfully bringing something fresh and natural inside, the energy of the sacred has entered into the kitchen.

Ingredients:

- 1 large handful of fresh herbs (i.e. basil, cilantro, parsley, mint, garlic chives)
- 1 handful of pumpkin seeds
- 1 tsp. of sea salt
- 1/2 tsp. nutritional yeast (optional for added cheesy flavor)
- 2 to 3 tbsp. of cold-pressed extra virgin olive oil

Directions:

Finely chop the herbs and seeds until combined and uniform in size. Add the sea salt (and nutritional yeast) to taste. Add the olive oil and mix. Enjoy immediately with gratitude.

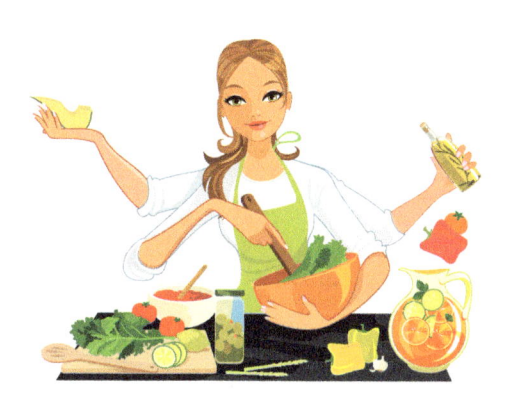

Cortney Chaite, CHC

Cortney is a certified weight loss coach, doTerra essential oils wellness advocate, Reiki-inspired energy worker, and Nia teacher. Cortney has a BA in art history from Vassar College, a master's of architecture from CUA and a certification in health coaching from the Institute of Integrative Nutrition. She is the founder of Cortney Chaite Coaching, where she guides women to reconnect with their inner magic through weight loss, self-love, and exploration of their inner passions. She offers individual programs designed to nourish the body, mind, and soul, as well as group detox and weight-loss programs.

- www.cortneychaitecoaching.com
- cortney@cortneychaitecoaching.com
- www.facebook.com/cortneychaitecoaching

PRACTICE 14

Love in the Kitchen

By Cortney Chaite, CHC

After years spent in architecture school gearing up for a career in design, I was blessed to have my first child. To say the least, it rocked my world. I soon found myself a stay-at-home-mom, full of love for my two children. I also found myself overweight, unhappy, sick, and suffering from a major loss of identity. As someone who was always highly energetic, enthusiastic, and full of life, I felt like I had disappeared and I was just going through the motions. I was existing, not living. My wakeup call came when my health started going downhill fast. I was having digestive problems, depression, dizziness, and extreme fatigue. I was too tired to play with my kids and I wasn't able to be the mother that I wanted to be.

As I hit rock bottom, I knew that I needed a major transformation. I wanted to get healthy, lose weight, and reconnect with myself again. Working with a health coach was pivotal for me. It became glaringly obvious that my relationship with myself had disappeared. I was living for everyone else and there was hardly any thought to what I needed to fuel my body and my soul. It was through this work that I started to reestablish what it meant to put myself first. I started to nourish my body, and my body came back to life. I started to nourish my passions, and my soul lit up. I didn't realize how much I had missed myself until I started to love myself again.

Today, I am the healthiest and strongest that I've ever felt. I also feel self-realized that I'm on the path to expressing my soul's true purpose. This transformation has had far-reaching consequences: my marriage is better, my friendships are better, my career is better, and my kids like having a happy, present, and healthy mom. None of this would have happened if I hadn't done some deep soul-searching and turned self-neglect into self-love. If there is one message that would distill the work that I do, it's to show yourself ruthless love, kindness, and gratitude. We can be so cruel to ourselves, yet we can love others with such reckless abandon our hearts feel like bursting. It is your job to learn to love yourself with that very same reckless abandon that you give to everyone and everything else.

It sounds so simple, but one of the most important and most effective ways to start showing ourselves kindness, gratitude, and love is through the food choices we make. This is where I started and where you can start, too. When transforming from a caterpillar into a butterfly, it's best to start with one thing at a time. How we feed ourselves can be one of the most loving choices we can make. Here's where to start: Make a list of all the reasons you want to improve your health or weight. As you're doing this, think of all the areas of your life that will improve if you were to reach your goals. Next, you can start creating consciousness around what you are eating by asking yourself, "Is this a loving choice for me?" Every time you eat something, you can also ask, "Will this help me reach my goals?"

As you take steps toward your health and happiness, you might find that you will learn to love food in a whole new way. Personally, I never wanted to admit that what I ate could impact my health. I was afraid I would lose a relationship with something that I loved dearly. However, once I started to change my diet, I had no idea that I could feel so *good*. Feeding myself became one of the new ways I learned to love myself, and it can be that way for you too.

It's amazing how powerful our minds are. In order to really implement this idea of self-love and self-kindness, you might have to break some pretty powerful habits. Most personal transformation programs last for approximately six months, so coaches can support clients as they create new and lasting habits. However, I'll share with you one of the most powerful tools you can implement to change your relationship with food: start praising yourself. Every time you make a loving decision, say, "Thank you." Every time you exercise, say, "You're such a badass!" If you find yourself caught in negative thinking, take a moment and try to notice the thoughts and endeavor to pick a more loving thought. You can even go as far as to write down the most common negative thoughts you use, then make a list of positive thoughts to replace them with. Keep this list with you and use it every time you catch yourself in a pattern of negative thinking.

After a while, the kindness you show yourself will catch up with you. You might find yourself looking forward to making positive choices because the payoff is love. Most of us will do anything for love. The more you learn to love yourself, the happier you will become. You will start to feel worthy of care and kindness. If you can practice showing your body gratitude, your body will love it! Once you embody the idea that you are worthy of your own love, you will radiate a new energy. You might find that your relationship improves, you get more respect at work, or people start to notice you in a new light.

They say that one drop creates a ripple effect. If your one drop is self-love and kindness, the ripples will reach to every area of your life. The ultimate gift for this hard work is simple and beautiful: you can stop being afraid of who you truly are, stand in your own skin, and love it.

ROASTED CHERRY TOMATOES, LEMON ZEST, SHALLOTS, GARLIC, AND OLIVE OIL

Ingredients:

- 24 oz. of mixed cherry tomatoes
- 1 1/2 tbsp. olive oil
- 2 large shallots, thinly sliced
- 2 garlic cloves, thinly sliced
- Zest of 1 small lemon
- 1/2 tsp. salt

Directions:

Preheat the oven to 400 degrees. Toss all the ingredients into a bowl and pour out onto a baking sheet. Roast in the oven for 40 minutes. Enjoy!

*These are delicious with any kind of meat or fish. You can make a large batch and store it in the fridge for a quick side dish. They're delicious warm or cold.

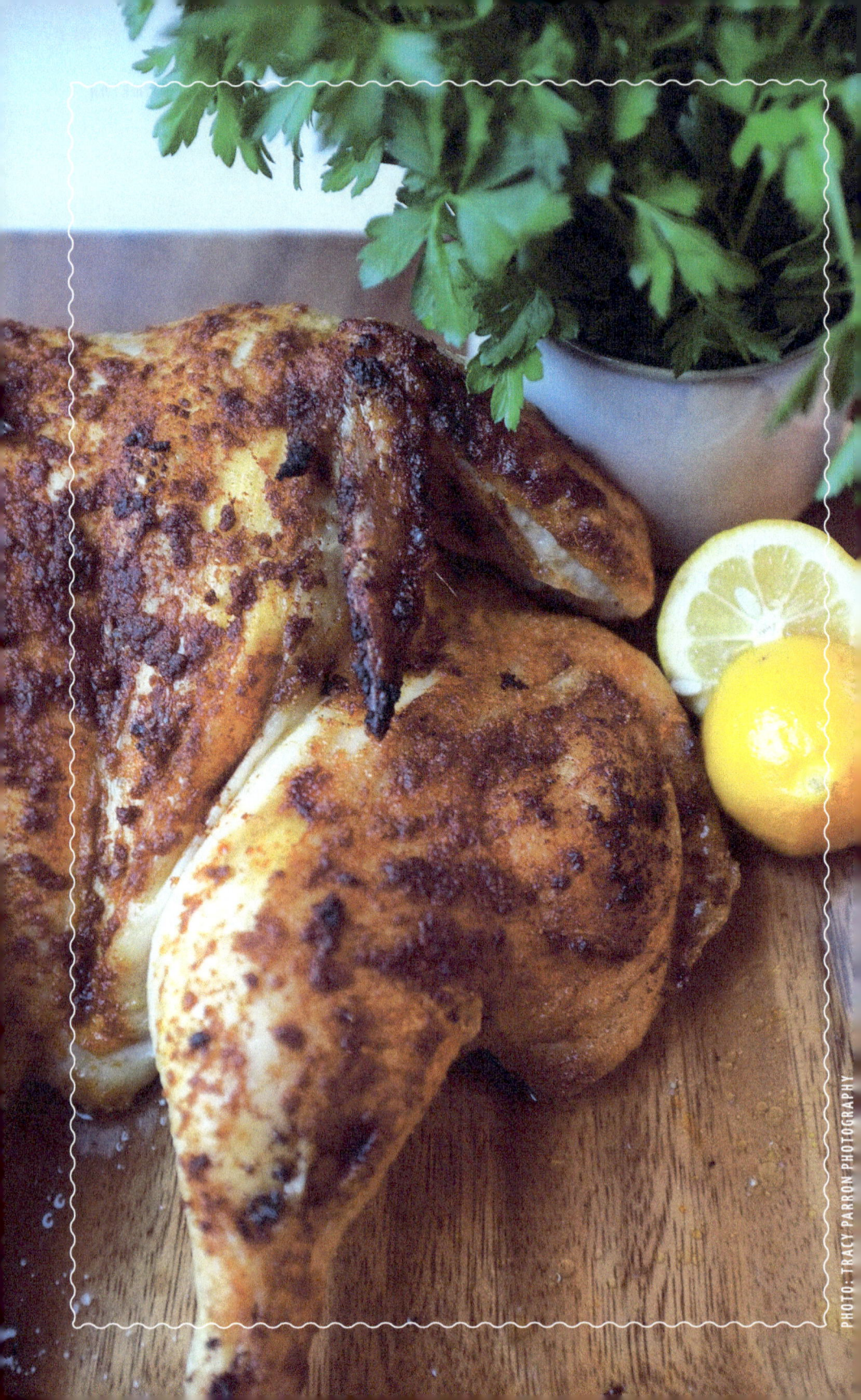

PHOTO: TRACY PARRON PHOTOGRAPHY

COMPILED BY **HEATHER EDEN**

SPATCHCOCKED CHICKEN WITH LEMON AND OLIVE OIL

Ingredients:

- 1 4 lb. whole organic (pasture raised if possible) chicken, spatchcocked (see instructions below)
- 1 lemon, juiced (about 1 tablespoon)
- 3 tbsp. olive oil
- 1 tsp. sea salt (approximate)
- 1 tsp. garlic powder (approximate)
- 1 tsp. sweet, smoked paprika (approximate)
- Black pepper to taste
- 1 large, yellow onion, sliced into 1/4 inch slices
- 1 lemon, sliced

Directions:

Preheat oven to 450 degrees. The easiest thing for a good spatchcock is to have your butcher do it! Saves time and trouble. If you'd like to do it yourself, get a pair of kitchen shears. Turn the chicken over so the breast side is down. You want to start cutting from the top of the chicken and cut toward the tail. Cut right along the backbone of the chicken, keeping as close to the bone as you can, first on one side and then the other. There might be a little resistance, but keep cutting! Once the backbone is removed, lay the chicken down with the breasts facing up. Time to get your hands dirty. You will push down on the breastbone until you hear it crack. Keep pushing down until your chicken lays open and flat. You can also Google, "How to spatchcock a chicken." You'll find some great tutorials. I highly recommend this before diving in!

Now that you've got a spatchcocked chicken, rinse with cold water and pat dry. Very dry. In a bowl, mix the lemon juice with the olive oil and rub this all over both sides of the chicken, making sure to get the skin fully covered. Sprinkle salt and pepper on the underside of the chicken and flip it over. Sprinkle the salt, garlic powder, and smoked paprika liberally all over the skin of the chicken. This will give the skin such delicious flavor, so don't leave any skin exposed!

Get a baking sheet and a wire rack. Slice the lemon and the onion and place on the baking sheet directly under where the chicken will rest. Lay the wire rack on top of the onions and lemon and place the chicken, skin side up, on the wire rack. Place the baking sheet on the middle rack in the oven and bake for 35 to 40 minutes for a 4 lb. chicken. When the internal temperature at the thickest part of the breast reads 165 degrees, you're done! Let the chicken rest for 10 minutes and enjoy!

COMPILED BY **HEATHER EDEN**

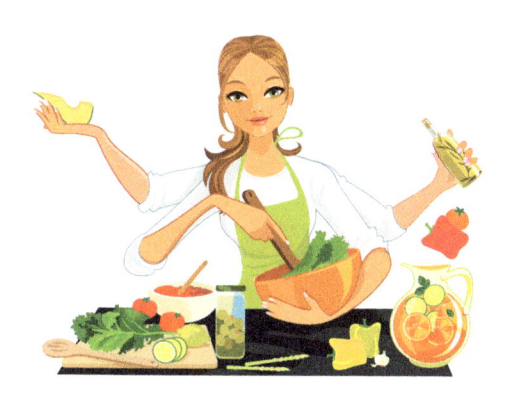

Tracey Camier, CHHC, AADP

Tracey Camier has over twenty years of cooking experience. In 2013, she received culinary training in the famous Napa/Sonoma Valley, CA. She earned her certification as a health coach from the Institute for Integrative Nutrition. Tracey creates many recipes using a whole food nutrition approach and is a passionate "healthy cooking" demonstrator in her community. She completed her BA at UW-Whitewater in psychology and has a background in social work, sales, and marketing. In 2012, she was awarded the Healthy Living Advocate of the Year from the YMCA of Metro Milwaukee. She is the founder of Arevitayou, LLC. Her coaching practice is built on revitalizing body, mind, and spirit through healthy lifestyle changes and strategies.

- www.Arevitayou.com
- Tracey.camier@arevitayou.com
- www.facebook.com/arevitayou

PRACTICE 15

Finding Acceptance with Food Allergies and Intolerances

By Tracey Camier, CHHC, AADP

I began an unexpected journey shortly after becoming a mom. My career and lifestyle plans changed after my oldest daughter was born. From the time she was a few days old, she developed rashes, skin, and breathing difficulties. These initial signs of food intolerance and allergies were worrisome and left us wondering what to do.

Apparently, what I was eating was affecting her, and by the time she was nine months old, skin-prick testing and trial and error determined that she was intolerant/allergic to dairy, eggs, soy, tree nuts, and peanuts. After receiving the results from this test, I chose to avoid these foods in my diet. For a period of time, even airborne food smells gave her severe reactions, like itchy rashes and wheezing. She lived solely on breast milk for eighteen months. (Needless to say, my desire to continue working with a successful career was put on hold in order for her to have a functional life.)

In time, I began to understand the difference between food allergies and intolerances. A food allergy is an exaggerated or unusual response to a food, caused by the body's immune system, which can cause serious illness or even death. Common allergens include tree nuts, peanuts, seafood, milk, and eggs. Checking all food labels is essential to avoiding possible allergens. Since 2004, the FDA acknowledged the need for disclosures and warnings on food packages. Labels now clearly state warnings such as "contains peanuts" or "manufactured in a facility that also processes tree nuts and peanuts."

Responses to food allergies often come on suddenly and can be triggered by just a small trace of the food. Reactions will occur every time the food is consumed. The reactions may continue to worsen and or they can be life threatening, as in the case of anaphylactic shock (Anaphylaxis) swelling of mouth, tongue, lips, wheezing, loss of blood pressure, chest pain. Other allergy responses include stomach pain, sneezing, diarrhea, hives, vomiting, itchy mouth, and dry cough. If an allergy is suspected, it is best to seek testing from a medical professional.

Food intolerances are becoming increasingly common (in Western diets) and are found more often than true allergies. Food intolerance or sensitivity occurs when a person has difficulty digesting a particular food. The reactions may be delayed, producing symptoms in one or more systems in the body. Symptoms generally develop gradually and may only manifest if the food is eaten often. Reactions are not life threatening and are often closely related to digestive issues. Some common reactions are headaches, bloating, mouth ulcers, body aches, and stomach or digestive issues.

One may not be aware of food intolerance until the food is eliminated from the diet for a period of two to four weeks and then reintroduced, noting any adverse reactions. Intolerance can result from the absence of vital enzymes needed to digest a food substance, along with sensitivity to food additives or reactions to naturally occurring chemicals in foods.

Around eighteen months of age, my daughter began eating pureed and followed with solid foods. She tolerated fruits and vegetables the best. Her favorite food became Futomaki (Maki) rolls. The Nori seaweed that is used to wrap the rolls is one of the food world's best sources of minerals. It contains protein, calcium, and vitamin C. I believe these foods are what helped heal my daughter's health. At around two years of age, she was referred to a pediatric dietician who informed me that my child's brain was not going to develop properly if I didn't give her larger quantities and a larger variety of foods. This rocked my world and began my journey into studying nutrition. I educated myself on enzymes and whole food nutrients. My daughter's chemistry, genetics, hormones, and her entire physiological makeup was different from every other child's. So, expecting her to eat and tolerate food like the next child was not realistic. I believe that due in large part to her getting the proper nutrients, her food intolerances diminished when she was just over two years old. Only a severe peanut allergy remains. She now eats a variety of nutritious whole foods and tries new things—with a little encouragement.

Having a loved one with a food intolerance and/or allergy can certainly be a big challenge. I discovered through the challenges that a lot of good came from it. My passion for cooking and gardening became part of my life again. Wanting to avoid allergens and cross-contamination from them spurred me on to prepare most of our meals and snacks at home. We avoid processed foods and labeled foods that have more than five ingredients. My family has gained a valuable conviction about the importance of eating nutritious foods that our bodies can digest, tolerate, and energize from.

My journey with foods has been the catalyst in seeking to become a Holistic Health Coach. Through the food and lifestyle changes I was able to implement as I studied, my husband discovered that he is hypoglycemic and I realized that I have food intolerances as well. We do our best to avoid the foods that trigger reactions and interfere with our ability to enjoy life fully. Cooking our own food, along with gardening and growing some of our food, has given us a new freedom! It is now my passion and heart's desire to help others gain a clear path to a healthier lifestyle, too.

I have the privilege of presenting healthy food demonstrations in my community. I truly enjoy creating original recipes using whole foods at the core. I teach others how to read labels and what to be aware of regarding food intolerances and allergies. In addition, I educate on how our bodies crave true nutrients and that cravings for processed foods diminish over time when whole, nutritious foods are a foundation in one's diet.

Obviously, taste is still of utmost importance when designing a recipe for frequent enjoyment. Here are two of my family's favorites. They are flavorful, easy to prepare, and of course, packed with nutrients! *Bon Appetit*!

BERRY MINESTRONE SURPRISE

Serves 4 to 8

Time: 10 minutes

Ingredients:

- 2 cups each of fresh strawberries, blackberries, blueberries, and raspberries
- 2 tbsp. cold water
- 3 tbsp. organic agave nectar
- 2 tsp. orange juice

Directions:

Wash and drain berries in a colander. Mix water, agave, and orange juice in large saucepan. Add strawberries, blackberries, and blueberries to saucepan and cook over a medium-low heat, bringing mixture to a slight boil. Stir gently and reduce heat to a simmer for 1 to 2 minutes. Let cool for 2 to 4 minutes. Gently mix in raspberries and serve.

Plating:

Place berry minestrone in a bowl and add a scoop of your favorite vanilla ice cream or frozen yogurt. Dairy-free options include coconut, almond, or soy ice cream. (For more flavor, zest a bit of orange to top the dish.)

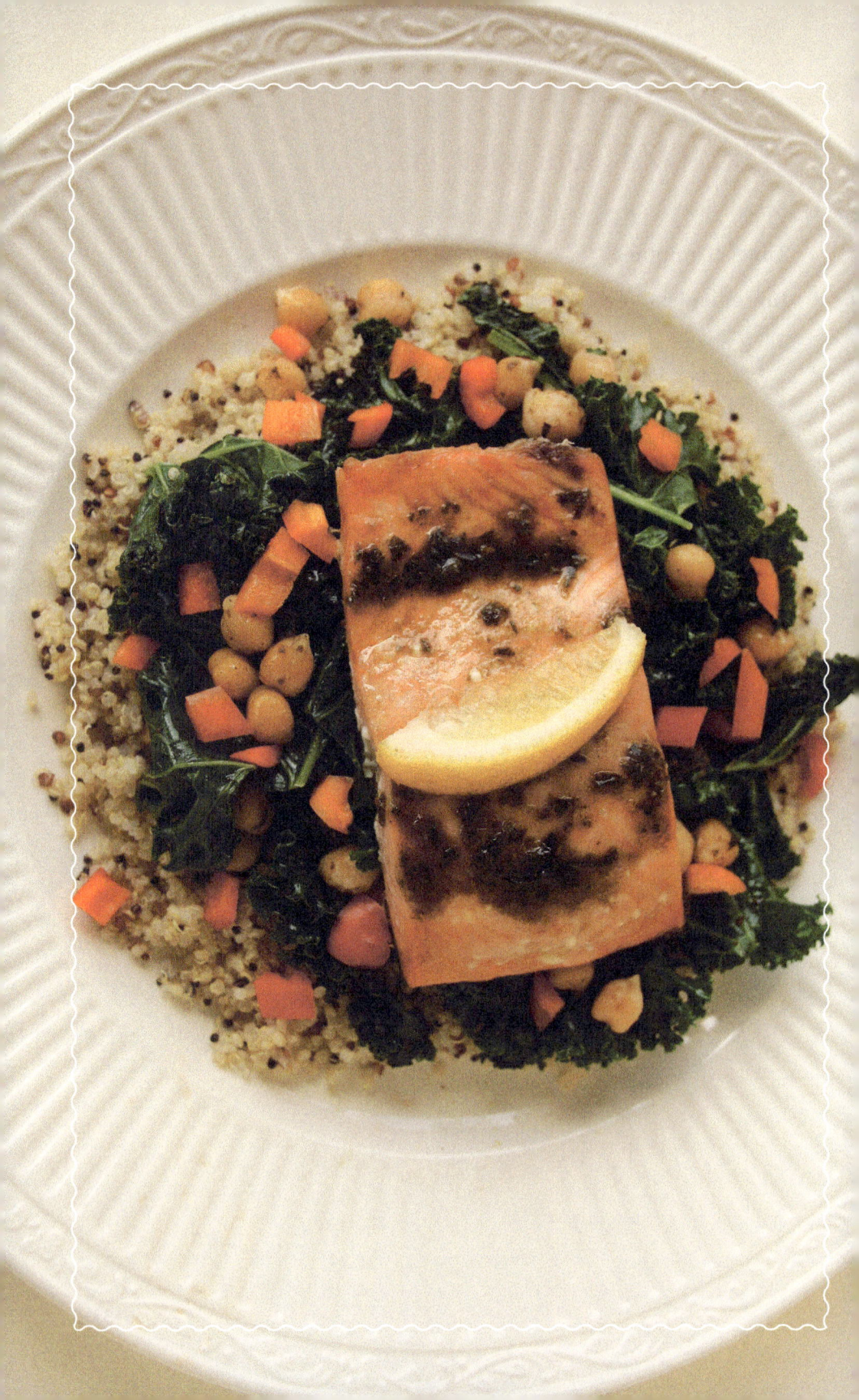

COMPILED BY **HEATHER EDEN**

BROILED SALMON OR CHICKEN OVER KALE PESTO QUINOA

Serves: 4 to 6

Time: 15 to 20 minutes

Ingredients:

- 1 to 2 cloves garlic
- 1/2 cup extra virgin olive oil
- 1/4 cup chickpeas, rinsed and drained (or pine nuts/walnuts for a more traditional pesto)
- 1/4 cup parmesan cheese, grated
- 3 cups fresh basil leaves
- 4 to 6 oz. of salmon fillets or chicken breasts
- 1 large bunch kale, chopped
- 2 (15 to 16 oz. cans) chickpeas, rinsed and drained
- 1 cup mixed sweet peppers, diced
- 1/2 lemon cut into 4 to 6 slices
- 1 to 2 cups of quinoa, rinsed and drained (can substitute brown or wild rice)
- Pinch of salt and pepper

Directions:

Measure 1 part quinoa to 1 1/2 parts water. Place in a medium saucepan, cover, and bring to a boil. Reduce heat and cook for 10 minutes. Stir and remove from heat. Keep covered for another 5 to 10 minutes.

Place fillets or chicken breasts (with a dash of pepper) on a broiling pan. Set oven temperature to low broil for 10 to 15 minutes.

Place olive oil, chickpeas (or nuts), garlic, parmesan cheese, and basil in food processor or blender. Blend sauce until a thin texture. Season with desired amount of sea salt and ground pepper.

Using a large sauté pan, add 3/4 of the pesto mixture. Cook over medium-low heat, adding kale and remaining chickpeas. Cover and sauté for approximately 5 minutes, stirring occasionally, until kale is slightly softened.

Plating:

Start with the quinoa then add the kale and chickpeas. Next, add diced peppers and top with the fillet. Drizzle the salmon or chicken with the rest of the pesto sauce. Top with freshly squeezed lemon.

COMPILED BY **HEATHER EDEN**

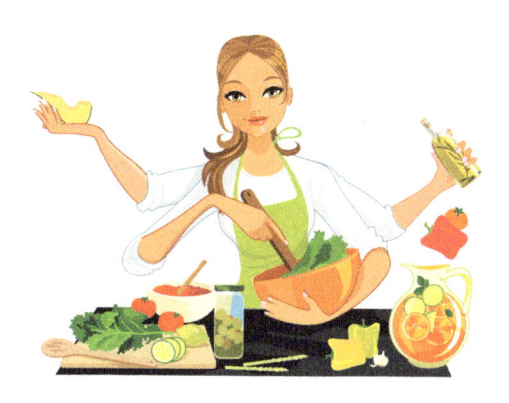

Michelle Grandy, CHHC, AADP, CRJCF, RYT

Michelle is a mother of three amazing sons, a wife, and a Certified Health Coach, Registered Yoga Teacher, Certified Facilitator, and Plant-Based Chef. She received her BS from Washington Adventist University. As a Health Coach, Michelle works with clients to uncover "core" causes of what's really holding them back from living a vibrant life. She enjoys supporting clients to reconnect with their body, mind, and spirit through nutrition and wellness. As a Certified Facilitator for the Canyon Ranch Institute, she plays an integral role in shaping the lives of the underserved and inner city local community, facilitating and teaching yoga, stress reduction, and meditation. Originally born and reared as a city girl in Washington, DC, Michelle has lived in Atlanta, GA, Syracuse, NY, and now resides in the Hilton Head, SC, area with her husband Albert, and two of her three sons, Albert III and Michael; her oldest son, Jamal is a young adult.

- www.ohhmichelle.com
- www.facebook.com/ohhmichelleom
- www.facebook.com/mtgrandy
- www.pinterest.com/ohhmichelle
- www.linkedin.com/in/ohhmichelle
- www.twitter.com/michelletgrandy

PRACTICE 16

Keeping a Balanced Body

By Michelle Grandy, CHC, AADP, CRICF, RYT

I can imagine people feeling overwhelmed by the confusing, often contradictory information around nutrition that floods social media and the like. Please don't let this curve your appetite in keeping a balanced body. Our thoughts, choices, and experiences influence our tendency to become either healthy or sick.

As a wife and a mother of three awesome sons, I have spent decades finding the divine in all endeavors. Through embracing a plant-based diet, I healed myself of what doctors insisted was an incurable ailment. This experience gave me a deeper connection to food, and proved to me the miraculous ability of the body to heal itself when supported with pure, whole, living foods. In keeping a balanced body, I enjoy empowering clients to make lasting health behavior changes that are cornerstones of lifelong wellbeing. I help to transform lives by teaching yoga and guiding clients on integrated nutrition, tweaking favorite foods, and substituting ingredients without compromising great taste!

I have always had a passion to change things and to inspire people to use their God-given gifts to make career-driven and business choices. I had been praying, for many years, asking God for His will over my life. I know I have a gift of giving and helping others but needed this to become more defined. My journey to becoming vegan was unexpected. I had read a book called *The Veganist*, by Kathy Freston, on my way to visit friends in California. I could not put the book down and had completed the book by the time the plane arrived in San Diego. In other words, I walked on the plane a carnivore and stepped off the plane a vegan!

Visiting California was a great place to begin my journey as a new vegan because there literally was a vegan-inspired restaurant on every corner. I had no idea how vegan food tasted and everything I knew about this vegan lifestyle, I learned within the five-hour plane ride. I didn't know what to eat, how to eat, or where to purchase food. I thought about my husband and boys and how this would change my family's entire mealtimes together. I hadn't even tasted anything vegan but was intrigued about how eating and consuming animal proteins had a direct effect on how my health, my asthma, my internal being, and how I look and feel. All I knew was that I wanted to change. I wanted to breathe normal again, on my own. I wanted not to depend on medications to make me feel better. I wanted to try this vegan lifestyle for myself to see if it would change my way of being…and oh boy, did it!

My first taste of a vegan meal was a "chick'n salad" sandwich, made of "mock" chicken. I was like, "What is that and what is mock chicken made of?" The sandwich was absolutely tasty! As a matter of fact, it was so good that I ate one every day for lunch that week as I learned what to eat and how to cook plant-based food. I immediately embraced and became empowered through research, reading science-based evidence articles, and reading books that would consume my thoughts and feed my soul about the vegan lifestyle. I started preparing meals, talking to other vegans, and tasting all kinds of vegan food. Whenever I travel, I make sure to visit a local vegan restaurant for taste, ideas, conversation, and resources. I am amazed at just how good eating a plant-based diet can be.

It has been more than five years since switching to a plant-based lifestyle. I didn't go vegan cold turkey because I wanted to lose weight or because I no longer wanted to contribute to the harm of animals. I became a vegan due to my health—asthma, to be more bold. I was born with asthma and have always been on the highest dosage of some sort of asthmatic medication, thereby taking medicine twice daily for a stronger, healthy heart, which came with a series of side effects. Today, I enjoy preparing all types of vegan dishes without compromising on great taste! It was one of the kindest decisions I could do for my body and the Universe.

What I do know for sure and what has worked for the family and me is to use these very simple yet easy-to-remember guidelines in sustaining and keeping a balanced body. First, I recommend you splurge on color,

color, and more color including red, purple, green, yellow, and blue vibrant colors of fruits and vegetables to nourish the body. Second, limit the white stuff—except for cauliflower, onions, and garlic—found in simple carbohydrates like white flour, white pasta, white rice, and white potatoes, since these do not regulate your blood sugar. Third, and after careful study, I typically do not recommend or eat anything my Grandmother Gussie didn't eat.

Modern food (today's food) that is sold is a far cry from the food my Grandmother Gussie ate, or the food our great-grandmothers had been eating since the dawn of time. Their food was naturally rich in whole grains, legumes, fruits, and vegetables, and I certainly don't remember eating processed foods, packaged foods, and very little junk food. Fourth, I suggest glancing at food labels, especially being cognizant of the first three or four ingredients, ensuring words like *sugar*, *sucrose*, *fructose*, or *high-fructose corn syrup* is not included. Fifth, buy local first, either from a Farmer's market or grocer who partners with local farmers. Six, I am a plant-based foodie eating, enjoying, and loving plant-based food. Plant-based food is less dense calorie-wise than animal-based food. It's loaded with vitamins, nutrients and fiber, in addition to being environmentally friendly—or ecofriendly. Last, never, *ever* skip breakfast. When in doubt, or pressed for time, mix whatever vegetables and fruit are on hand—some nuts and seeds, and nondairy milk or water—and add them to a blender to satisfy your first meal of the day.

I am often in a frenzy in the morning, gathering stuff, getting my boys ready for school, packing lunches, and making sure my husband is cared for. I thrive from the choice of having handy a wide variety of plant-based ingredients, including choosing vegetables and herbs from the backyard vertical aeroponic tower garden. I often send my sons out to grab vegetables and herbs to throw in the blender to mix a green smoothie for everyone as breakfast.

I certainly understand the power of keeping a balanced body through consuming healthy foods and quieting the mind and body, to reconnect with breath through practicing yoga every day, not just for myself, but through educating my family, friends and community on the need to stay cognitively balanced with food and movement.

CREAMY AND CHUNKY CURRY CHICKEN SALAD (VEGAN)

Ingredients:

- 1 package soy chicken nugget, non-breaded (Non-GMO), diced
- Fresh bunch of spinach
- 1 cup nondairy mayonnaise
- 1/4 cup onion, chopped
- 1/4 cup celery
- 2 tbsp. ground curry powder – or more to taste
- 1 tsp. dried chives
- 1 tsp. dried parsley
- 1 tsp. dried thyme
- 1 tsp. onion powder
- 1 tsp. garlic powder
- 1 tsp. cilantro
- 1 tsp. sea salt
- 1 tsp. black pepper
- 1/2 tsp. red pepper flakes
- 1 tsp. paprika

Directions:

Combine all ingredients well, sprinkle with dried parsley, refrigerate, and serve

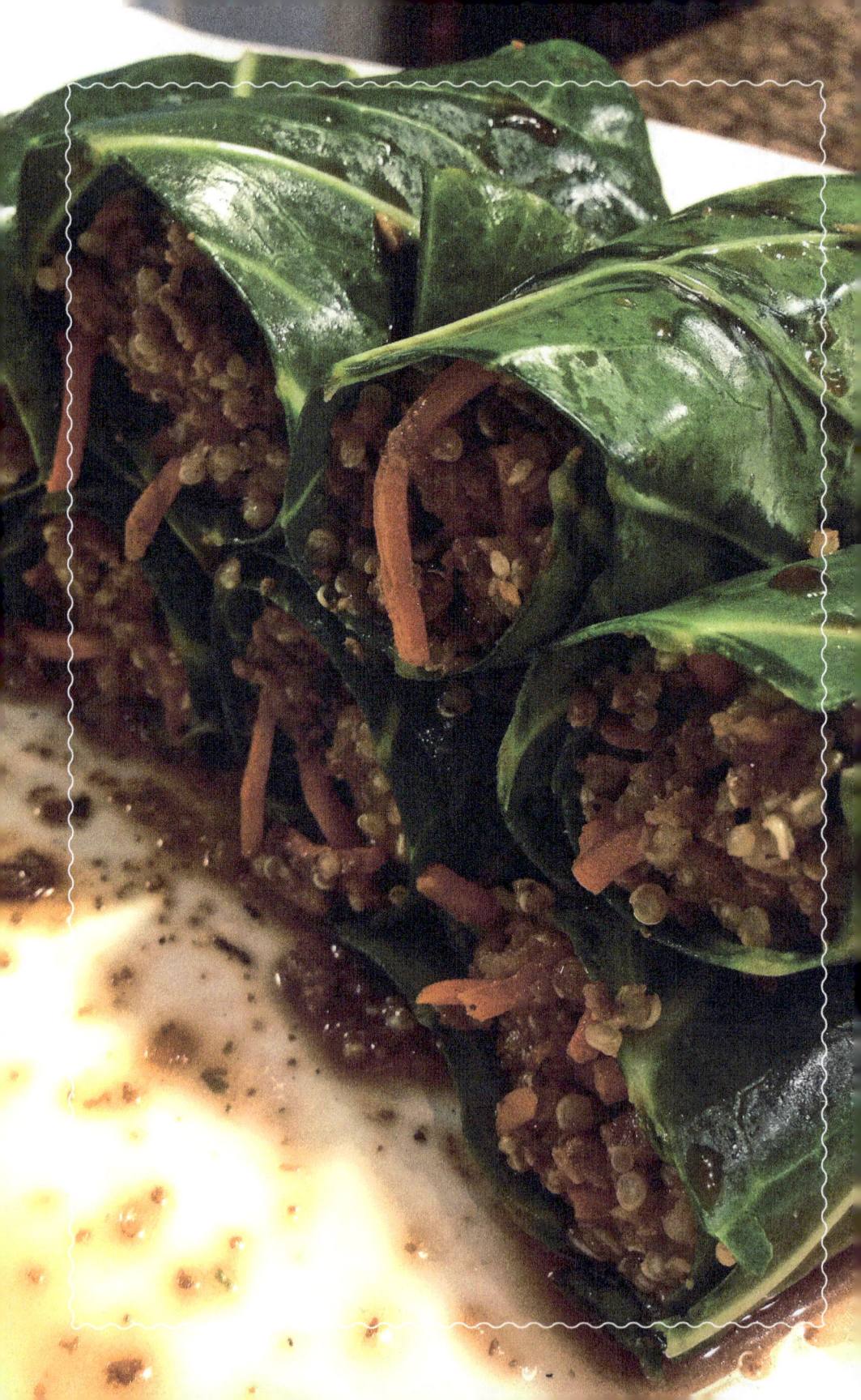

STUFFED COLLARDS WRAP (VEGAN)

Ingredients:

FILLING

- 1 pound meatless crumbles
- 1 1/2 tbsp. coconut oil
- 2 cloves garlic, minced
- 1 large onion, chopped
- 2 stalks celery, chopped
- 2 medium carrots, chopped
- 1 cup "no chicken" broth (found in organic section of grocer) or vegetable broth
- 1/4 tsp. cayenne pepper
- 1 tsp. basil
- 1 tsp. thyme
- 1 cup cooked quinoa
- 1/4 cup chopped fresh parsley leaves
- 1 bunch collard greens, about 12 leaves, stalks discarded
- Sea salt and pepper to taste

MARINADE

- 1/3 cup freshly squeezed orange juice
- 3 tbsp. tamari sauce
- 1 clove garlic, minced
- 3 tbsp. rice vinegar

Directions for marinated collards:

Cut or pull greens away from stem, keeping greens in large pieces. Place collards in large bowl and mix well with marinated sauce ingredients (above). Carefully transfer 12 large leaves to a baking sheet lined with paper towels.

Directions for collards filling:

Heat oil in a heavy-bottomed sauté pan over medium-high heat.

Add the meat crumbles, and brown. Add garlic, onion, celery, carrots, basil, and thyme.

Cook for about 3 minutes. Season with salt and pepper to taste.

Add the no-chicken broth, or vegetable broth, and cayenne. Stir in the cooked rice and parsley, mixing thoroughly, letting the broth reduce until there is no moisture left in the pan.

Arrange a reserved collard leaf on your work surface and top with 1/3 cup rice filling. Roll up, starting with the large end of the leaf and rolling it over the filling, tucking in the ends like a burrito. Repeat with remaining leaves and filling, and serve.

COMPILED BY **HEATHER EDEN**

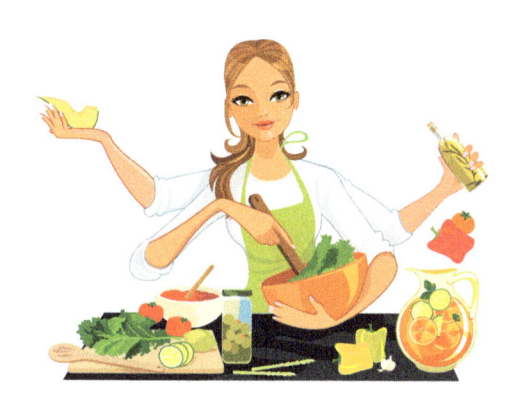

Abby Phon, CHHC, AADP, IAHC

Abby Phon is a certified holistic health and wellness coach. She received her training at the Institute for Integrative Nutrition in New York City. She is certified by the American Association of Drugless Practitioners and is a member of the International Association for Health Coaches. Abby leads corporate workshops on nutrition and lifestyle, conducts food tours, cooking demonstrations, and offers individual health and nutrition coaching around the world. Abby is a regular contributor for the health and wellness website, MindBodyGreen. Her recipes and articles have been published globally by Conscious Divas, Cafe Truth, All Things Healing, EatSmart Products, and more. Abby is also a Beauty Ecologist for Pangea Organic Skincare and a distributor for Young Living Essential Oils.

- www.feedyourmindbodyspirit.com
- www.facebook.com/AbbyPhon
- www.twitter.com/AbbyPhon
- www.pinterest.com/abbyphon
- www.pangeaorganics.com/abbyphon

PRACTICE 17

Healthy Sugars

By Abby Phon, CHHC, AADP, IAHC

Do you have a sweet tooth? Do your kids? It's hard not to! Sugary snacks and treats are all over the place, with colorful wrappers and cartoon mascots. Plus, as a busy mom, when we're pressed for time and need a quick pick-me-up (or stressed out and overwhelmed and need an emotional boost), sugar is there at the ready. Our bodies are prewired to treat sugar as a reward. Have you ever caught yourself bribing your kids to finish their dinner by offering dessert? It totally works!

I LOVE candy! Or at least I used to. My sister likes to remind me that as a child, I could hear candy being unwrapped a mile away, and come running.

But there's a downside. Not only are there the obvious maladies (sugar rush, sugar crash cycles, and/or tooth decay), but many subtle and seemingly unrelated ailments can be traced directly back to sugar!

I'm a recovering drug addict, but it's not what you think. As a child, I suffered from severe allergies. Although I didn't (nor did my parents) realize it at the time, this was exacerbated by my overconsumption of sugar (along with not being breastfed—but that's another story for another time!). I was on allergy pills every single day (multiple pills a day), took steroids, inhalers for asthma, and received allergy shots a few times a week. I was on drugs my entire life. And I STILL had bad allergies!

That experience left me really distrustful of Western medicine and its over-reliance on pills and shots. As a young adult, while going through a hard divorce, instead of prescriptions and pills, I turned to sugar. I would eat my emotions and try to mend my broken heart with pints and pints and pints of frozen yogurt. In one memorable incident, I went to Whole Foods (in tears and pj's!) and bought six pints of FroYo. I ate that all in two days. I would go through a few packages of chocolate chips each week—and that doesn't even include the packages of Twizzlers, Swedish Fish, and other candy, sorbet, or frozen yogurt I could get my hands on. Since weight wasn't a problem for me, I thought my sugar consumption binges were perfectly healthy and normal. And then it hit. I couldn't move. Literally. I was exhausted for weeks, months…I felt like I was eighty years old! I was SO tired and getting sick often (with colds and bronchitis). I finally got sick of feeling sick and tired and did something about it. From my earlier experience, I wanted to find a way without drugs (or Western doctors who continued to prescribe them).

I started learning about what sugar really does to you and your body, and realized I had to make a drastic shift. By cutting out the processed and refined sugars, I really noticed a difference. Today, I am allergy-free, full of energy, and I feel so much better and have a much healthier attitude towards my food and nourishment.

Sugar suppresses the immune system. When you eat a big dose of sugar, like a soda or a candy bar, you temporarily suppress your immune system's ability to respond to challenges. The effect lasts for several hours, so if you eat sweets several times a day, your immune system may be really struggling. Sugar also promotes inflammation, which contributes to aging and disease.

Besides leading to inflammation and suppressing the immune system, sugar can cause fatigue and diseases like diabetes, heart disease, asthma, allergies, IBS, obesity, eczema, and the list goes on!

When was the last time you read the label on your favorite box of "healthy cereal?" Know what's in your food: READ THE LABEL! Ingredients are listed in order of quantity. Sometimes there are several kinds of sugar—corn syrup, sugar, dextrose, fructose, maltose…the list goes on. If you added them all together, it might very well be the number one ingredient.

So what can you do about it? You can "crowd out" sugary foods by adding in more green vegetables, whole grains, and other filling and healthy foods. If you need to sweeten things up, try some healthier alternatives to white sugar.

Natural sweeteners are things like: honey, dates, maple syrup, organic raw agave, coconut sugar, molasses, and fruit. They usually either contain vitamins and minerals along with the sweetness, or have a lower glycemic index, which makes them easier on your body. The best alternatives? Low-sugar fruit and sweet vegetables.

Here is something you can teach your children: healthy foods are good for you and nourishing but can still satisfy that innate sweet tooth every child seems to have! What do I mean? Long before food processing, the only source of sweet tastes were plant foods, like whole grains, root vegetables (like sweet potato, carrots, and parsnips), other vegetables, and fruit. So in order to get the sweet taste the body desired, people had to eat plants! And it's no coincidence that these sweet foods are also great sources of nutrients, energy, and fiber.

I love the challenge and creativity of creating recipes (and adapting old ones!) to make it healthier for my family. I literally don't have any white sugar in the house and I rarely buy any processed prepackaged foods. Another advantage of making your own sweet treats is just that—if you don't have it in the house, you won't eat it! And if you go to the trouble of cooking something up, you'll care more about what goes in it and usually choose healthier ingredients and feel good about what you're eating!

I'm not a big proponent of deprivation. I don't think that results in lasting, meaningful changes in your life. What I really endorse is channeling your cravings and desires into healthier choices that still satisfy that taste or flavor or sensation you were looking for. I think it's super important to start this process young.

So here's your chance to break the cycle before it starts! Help your children discover that sweet and delicious tastes don't always come wrapped in cellophane. My recipe below for a Spring Mint Pea Puree is full of nutrition and healthy carbohydrates but still sweet enough to satisfy that sugar craving. And when you really need a treat, my vegan strawberry "ice cream" gives you all the flavor without the refined white sugar or high-fat cream. Both of these recipes are easy ways to get your kids involved in the kitchen and show them how real ingredients turn into healthy and delicious food!

As a mom, I'm all about simple and quick, but that doesn't have to mean unwrapping takeout or nuking something prepackaged. There are so many delicious and nutritious things you can do in just a few minutes with real whole foods! When you're really in a bind, a good blender or food processor is amazing. In minutes, you can have soups, smoothies, dips, spreads, mousses, sorbets, and other desserts. Check out these two easy recipes to get you started!

In good health,

Abby

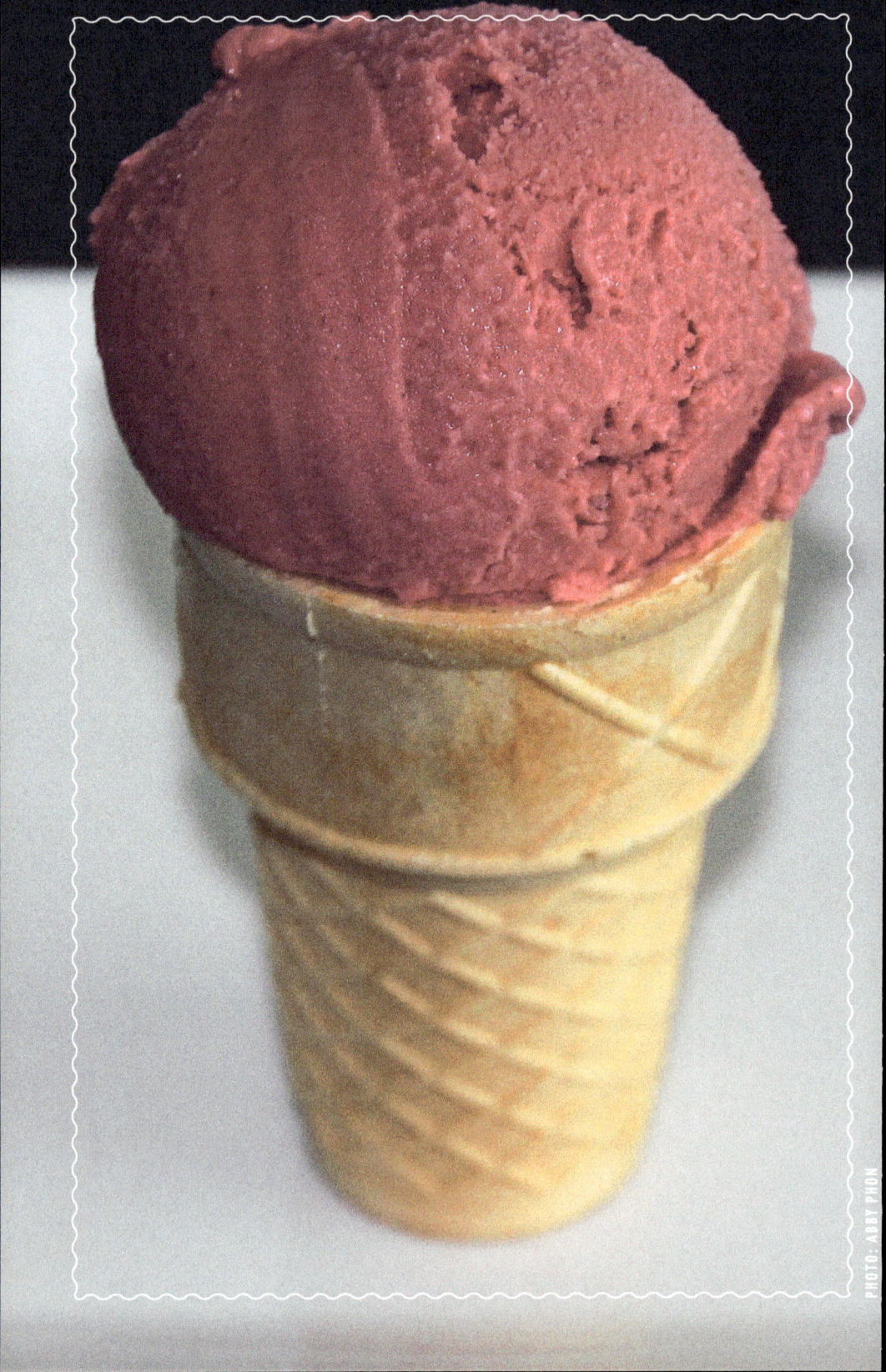

VEGAN STRAWBERRY ICE CREAM

For my daughter's birthday, I had a small party and made an impromptu pink-themed menu, and this strawberry vegan ice cream was a huge hit.

It's a healthy and refreshing treat that doesn't sit as heavy as its dairy frozen counterpart. For a fun flair, I put a scoop into an ice cream cone. Perfect and healthy for kids of all ages!

Agave is definitely a sugar, but raw organic agave has a lower glycemic index than other simple sugars. This means it's absorbed into your bloodstream more slowly, letting your body adjust and digest it without a sugar rush (or crash.) Be careful when you buy it though, since some of the cheaper brands are highly refined and really no better than corn syrup! You could always substitute maple syrup or date honey!

Ingredients:

- 1 cup raw organic cashews, soaked in water overnight
- 4 cups frozen organic strawberries
- 3/4 cup raw organic agave (or to taste)

Directions:

Drain the cashews. Add the cashews, strawberries, and agave to a Vitamix or blender. Blend until smooth. Freeze for about an hour to firm up to an "ice cream" texture.

Note: if you freeze this longer, take it out to soften before serving. It freezes quite solid.

SPRING MINT PEA PUREE

Serves about 6 to 8

This dish is super versatile. Experiment and have fun! It's delicious and healthy, and because the peas are naturally sweet it helps reduce your kids' cravings for sweet treats after the meal! Here are a few suggestions to get you started:

- Serve lamb chops or salmon over it—great as a side dish!
- Serve on crostini or rice crackers as an elegant and vivid appetizer.
- Add water, veggie broth or almond milk for a fresh soup.
- Toss with your favorite pasta and garnish with fresh basil for a light Italian twist!
- Does double-duty as baby food!

Ingredients:

- 2 cups fresh spring peas or 16 oz. frozen organic petite peas
- 4 sprigs organic fresh mint
- 1 clove garlic, minced
- 1 tbsp. extra virgin olive oil
- 1/2 tsp. sea salt
- 1/4 tsp. black pepper

Directions:

If using frozen peas, pour boiling water over them to defrost. Add peas, garlic, salt, pepper, and oil to food processor and blend. Add the fresh mint and blend again until well mixed. Serve however you like! (See suggestions above). Garnish with a small sprig of fresh mint!

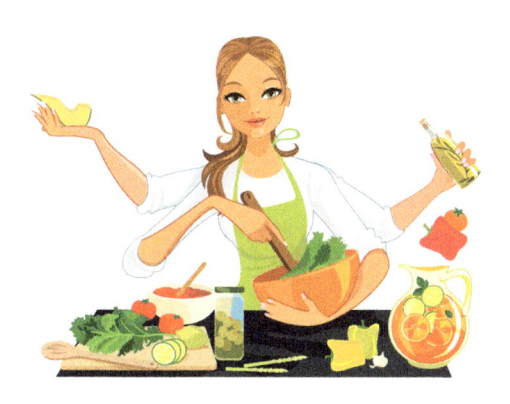

Diane Hoch, CHC

Diane Hoch is a certified nutritional health counselor, natural foods chef, and founder and CEO of The Food Evolution. She is a gluten-free and dairy-free chef committed to sharing nutrition education to children and parents, and is a crusader for better school food. Diane believes in natural foods as a source of preventative medicine, and her mission is to spread the message of "whole foods" nutrition through private counseling, cooking classes, and educational nutrition videos. She also works among The Rockland Coalition for Better School Food, The Rockland Farm Alliance, and The Rockland County School Health and Wellness Coalition.

PRACTICE 18

Finding Happiness through Non-judgment

By Diane Hoch, CHC

We all experience points in our lives where we are taught that it is wrong to judge others, but I've come to realize that the most painful of judgments come from judging ourselves. Whether it is carried from childhood to adulthood, or from ongoing judgments placed upon us by others, judging is destructive and doesn't serve any positive purpose. So why is it that we are so hard on ourselves? How can we move from a place of criticism to places of motivation, comfort, and supportive behaviors?

When it comes to food, we are in such a transitional and confusing time. The media bombards us with fast, frozen, and processed food choices that are marketed to us with the promise of making our lives easier. Our intuition tells us that eating wholesome, real foods that come from the earth is the healthier option. Following our intuition is part of the process of developing a healthier lifestyle and that is why you are reading this book. There is a simple, intuitive process if you want to start cooking healthier for your family. The process begins when you stop judging yourself for what you are not doing and congratulate yourself for making the decision of wanting to add healthier choices into your weekly recipes. Just like that, you're already moving forward.

You are a caring, loving, and nurturing mother who wants the best for her family. At times of judgment, it is easy to feel insecure about your parenting abilities, and this will cause you to feel isolated and self-conscious about your fears. This is where I want to remind you to stop being so hard on yourself and take a deep breath, because it's not as difficult as you may think! Briefly reflect on other challenges you've endured and say "I have been here before, and I will definitely get through this!" In the moment, things always appear worse than they are, and that's because we add judgment to the situation and cause it to escalate out of proportion. Relax, reflect, and you'll make strides.

I often tell people to meet themselves where they are, and I do believe this to be a powerful and empowering statement. In order to meet yourself where you are, it is important to stop judging yourself based on where you may be. Food is often used as an emotional crutch, and certain foods are the perfect pitfall for stressful times in our lives. Our stress eating leads us to consuming the "comfort foods" we were raised on. They are usually choices that are addictive, sugar-laden detriments to our health. Raising kids is not always easy — I happen to have three teenage daughters, so I can relate to many stressful moments along the way. The thing we seem to forget in those moments of stress is that we are all human beings on a journey through life, and none of us are perfect! Truthfully, what fun would that be anyway?

It seems the older I get, the more I realize that we are all similar in that we need to practice being nonjudgmental towards both ourselves and others. I do believe that we were brought into a world of judgments. I personally grew up with a long list of what I call "should-be's." My siblings and I were expected to adhere to a long list of requirements such as: be well behaved at all times, be dressed a certain way for school and family functions, have our elbows off the table. And if you stepped out of line for just a moment in public — oh my goodness! As much as I value good manners and proper etiquette, I believe that many of these expectations began our relationship with self-judgment, and consequentially, the judgment of others. How can children learn from a scolding? What did that teach us? If we didn't adhere to proper behaviors, were we less worthy of affection and respect? Were we supposed to look at others who behaved differently and consider them "less-than" or beneath us? Think about these things as you are raising your own children — what is really important when all is said and done? I believe it is to love, honor, and respect both yourself and your family — especially your children.

If we look at the airbrushed images of how girls and women are portrayed in magazines today, it might give you some indication of the pressure we are under around body image. Being able to observe how critical the world can be though the lens of my children gave me a keen sense of awareness into this harsh reality. Although my experience is with girls, I can say that boys certainly feel the pressure of judgment just the same. Food and judgment go hand in hand today. If you are overweight, you are being judged, and if you are underweight, you are being judged. Eating health-supportive, home-cooked, whole foods with your family will support them in so many ways. Teaching these lifelong habits and having delicious and nutritious foods as your families "comfort foods" will be a gift that will continue supporting them throughout their entire lives. The ripple effect will carry down to future generations, as well. This is the mission I represent in my nutrition and cooking center, The Food Evolution, as well as my personal lifestyle.

So how do we best support ourselves in this difficult world of judgment we live in? Well, the good news is that there are certainly many ways, and the foods we choose to eat can be a major source of comfort and support. I encourage you to find the time to create the recipes that I have shared with you in this book, my other cookbooks, and cooking videos. I hope that you share this wonderful food with those you love and continue to practice self-love and non-judgment for your own self and those around you!

CRISPY GARLIC, SPINACH AND CHICKPEA BURGERS WITH AVOCADO

Ingredients:

- 4 cups cooked chickpeas
- 2 avocados
- 2 cups spinach, chopped
- 1 cup carrots, shredded
- 3/4 cup garbanzo bean flour
- 1/2 cup red onion, diced
- 3 tbsp. garlic, minced
- 2 tbsp. olive oil
- 2 tbsp. chia seeds and 6 tbsp. water*
- 1 tsp. turmeric
- 1 tsp. cumin
- 1 tbsp. sea salt
- 1/2 tsp. pepper

Olive Oil and Garlic Mixture:

- 3 tbsp. olive oil
- 2 tbsp. fresh garlic, pressed

Directions:

Preheat oven to 375 degrees.

*To prepare chia seed mixture, add chia seeds to water and set to the side. After 5 to 6 minutes, whisk and the mixture will become gelatinous.

In a large sauté pan over medium heat, add olive oil and cook onions and garlic until translucent, about 5 minutes. Add carrots, spinach, turmeric, cumin, and continue cooking until carrots are soft, about 3 to 5 minutes. Turn off heat and set pan aside. In a food processor, pulse the chickpeas until mostly smooth leaving about 1/3 in a chunky texture.

Here is the rest of this recipe:

Add chickpeas to sauté pan with vegetables and mix to deglaze and combine before transferring to a large bowl.

Fold in chia seed mixture well before adding garbanzo bean flour, salt and pepper.

Shape mixture into burger form and place on parchment lined baking sheet.

Create your Olive Oil & Garlic mixture topping by combining the 3 Tablespoons Olive Oil and 2 Tablespoons pressed Garlic – then use this to spoon a dollop on top of the burgers and spread to coat. Bake in oven for 10 minutes. Remove, flip, and return to oven for additional 15 minutes.

Turn oven to Broil at 450 degrees and finish cooking to create a golden brown topping.

Place burger on plate and top with sliced Avocado. Serve and Enjoy! Yum!

COMPILED BY **HEATHER EDEN**

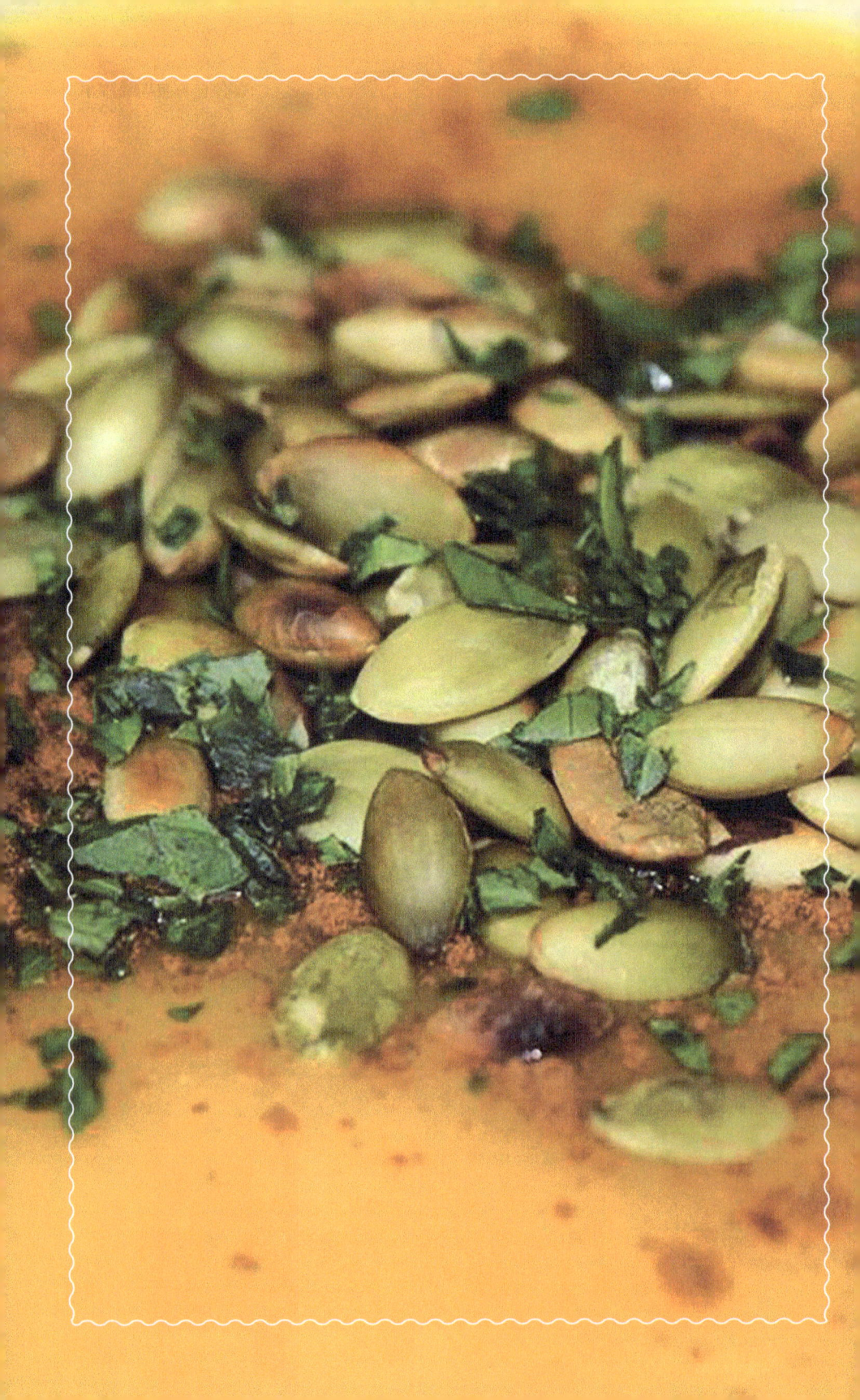

BUTTERNUT SQUASH AND RED LENTIL SOUP WITH CINNAMON

Ingredients:

- 1 large butternut squash (approx. 6 cups), peeled, seeded, and cubed
- 8 cups low sodium vegetable broth
- 3 tbsp. olive oil
- 3 cups white onions, diced
- 1 tsp. ginger, ground
- 1 tsp. sea salt
- 1/2 tsp. black pepper
- 1 1/2 cups red lentils
- 8 tbsp. toasted pumpkin seeds (pepitas)*
- Chopped parsley to taste
- 2 tsp. cinnamon, ground

Directions:

In a soup pot, sauté onions with olive oil over medium heat until translucent, 3 to 4 minutes. Add butternut squash cubes, ginger, salt, and pepper. Cook, stirring often for an additional 3 minutes.

Add the broth and lentils to the pot. Bring to a boil then reduce heat, cover, and simmer for 30 minutes. Use an immersion blender to puree the soup until smooth. For a thicker consistency, allow soup to cook uncovered over a low boil, stirring occasionally.

Ladle soup into bowls and sprinkle with cinnamon, toasted pumpkin seeds, and chopped parsley.

*In a medium sauté pan, over medium heat dry toast the pumpkin seeds until they begin to puff and turn slightly brown, approximately 2 to 3 minutes. Remove immediately from heat and place in serving dish.

COMPILED BY **HEATHER EDEN**

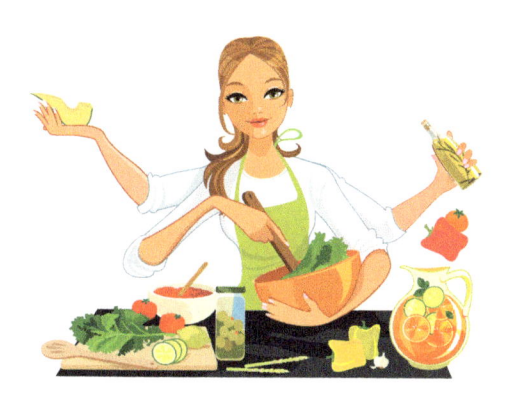

Robin Von Schwarz, CHHC, AADP, RYT

Robin is a certified holistic health coach and yoga teacher, specializing in neuro-nutrient therapy and restorative yoga for anxiety and depression. She has a BS degree in journalism with a minor in English from Texas A&M University-Commerce, and has taught high school English, speech, and AVID. After watching her own children and many of her students suffer with anxiety and depression, she resigned from teaching, became certified as a health coach through the Institute for Integrative Nutrition, and founded Hunger4Healing Holistic Health Coaching, LLC. It is her mission to educate young people about their physical and mental health.

- www.Hunger4Healing.com
- www.facebook.com/pages/Hunger4Healing/331588640283715#
- robin@hunger4healing.com
- www.hunger4healing.idlife.com
- @hunger4healing
- www.twitter.com/Hunger4Healing

PRACTICE 19

The Health Benefits of Being Present

By Robin Von Schwarz, CHHC, AADP, RYT

A child's nutritional, physical, emotional, mental, and spiritual health work interdependently and are influenced by the health of the family unit. Unfortunately, in the chaotic world we live in today, it seems as if we don't have time to focus on the state of our families. We are rushing from one event to another and the family has taken a backseat to individual pursuits, limiting our time to cook healthy meals, communicate, and just be present. Subsequently, the fast-paced culture we live in is compromising the overall health of our children. Childhood obesity and disease are on the rise, mental health issues are more prevalent than ever before, social media is dictating morality, and kids are emotionally disconnected.

As a young mom of four children, three who are grown and on their own now, I was committed to making my families' health a priority. I had practiced good nutrition for several years prior to having babies, so it was natural for me to eat healthy while I was pregnant, birth each of my kids naturally, and nurse them, giving them the best start in life I knew how to give. When my children were old enough to be given responsibility, they took part in mealtime preparations, and we always sat down together. I knew it was important to make mealtime a family event. Unfortunately, as my children got older, I allowed our family's health to be dictated by ballgames, piano lessons, and even church activities. We started eating on the run and making poor food choices. If I managed to cook a complete meal, my focus changed from promoting family time to finishing as quickly as possible.

During those years when life seemed to be more about getting everything done versus living in the moment, I discouraged my kids when they wanted to help cook dinner. My youngest son often asked if he could help, but most of the time I put him off, because it was quicker to do things myself. In retrospect, I wish I'd slowed down and taken those seemingly insignificant moments more seriously. These are the moments that count. These are the moments that tell our kids they are important to us, that we have time for them, and that we are really listening. Those moments provide us the opportunity to model healthy habits in all areas of our kids' lives.

For many years, I took my children's physical, mental, and emotional health for granted. As far as I knew, I was doing a great job and I was in control. I bought fresh veggies and fruit from a local family farm, juiced carrots and apples here and there, belonged to a whole foods co-op, taught Sunday school, and was a room mom at the school. Little did I know then that I was only in control of my day-to-day choices. More often than not, we are not in control of what happens to us but only how we respond to what happens. So, when my oldest daughter nearly died from a ruptured ovarian cyst at age ten, I started looking more closely at my daily choices. I started paying attention to the hormones that are added to our meat and dairy, researched the local water, stopped using plastic in the microwave, and anything else I thought might have caused her body to be out of balance.

It was just three years later that the same daughter stopped functioning normally because of debilitating obsessive-compulsive disorder, or OCD. I didn't see it coming. I had to become an expert on OCD, researching the brain, and becoming familiar with terms like *neurotransmitter function* and *frontal lobe activity*. I learned more about how our diets affect our mental health. It took three years, but my daughter overcame her OCD without the medications her doctors told me she would need to take the rest of her life. Unfortunately, it wasn't long after she recovered that my oldest son became depressed and suicidal after the sudden death of a close friend. Through both my daughter's illnesses and my son's six-year fight against depression, it was my faith that sustained me.

I wanted to help my son, my daughter, and others who suffered from similar illnesses related to anxiety and depression, so I went back to school to become a holistic health coach. I began to unravel the connections between diet and proper neurotransmitter functions. I was introduced to the term *epigenetics* and learned that while we might have certain inherited genes that predispose us to illness, we also have the power to turn those genes on or off by the choices we make.

Becoming healthy is a process. Being aware of what we put into our bodies, our hearts, and our minds is a practice in awareness. Learning to be present with our children and with our family members is critical to everyone's emotional health and mental wellbeing. You won't get it all right over night, but you have to begin. I began by unlearning all I thought to be true. Then I stopped buying processed, chemically-laden foods and removed them from my home. I stopped going to fast food restaurants. I learned about addictive foods. Unfortunately, many of those foods, like dairy, I believed were good for my family. And I began to understand how important it is to take care of my own physical and emotional health so that I can be an example for my children. Children mirror what they see. And my children were seeing a stressed out mom. What do your children see when they look at you?

The recipes I am sharing are vegan, but not because I believe everyone should be vegan. I do, however, believe in eating clean meats and doing so in moderation. It takes very little meat to meet our daily protein requirements. There is a connection between mental illness and inadequate protein intake, so being vegan is a decision that should only be made if someone is taking the proper precautions. You must make sure to get enough protein through the ingestion of greens, nuts, and legumes. Both of my recipes provide adequate protein.

I chose to include my Tex-Mex Vegan Chili because it goes against some preconceived notions that vegan food is bland and boring! The second recipe I chose is Vegan Shepherd's Pie. It is great when warm "comfort food" is desired. My non-vegan kids love both recipes. Becoming healthy has brought my family closer together. Once again, mealtime is a time to share and be present with those I love.

VEGAN SHEPHERD'S PIE WITH CASHEW GRAVY

Ingredients:

- 24 oz. organic veggie crumbles
- 4 to 5 cups cooked mashed yams (3 to 4 large yams)
- 1 1/2 large diced onions
- 6 cups fresh spinach
- 7 to 10 oz. frozen mixed peas, corn, and carrots
- 1 to 2 cups fresh organic cashews (soak overnight prior to use).
- 1 tsp. fresh garlic
- Sea salt, white pepper, chili powder
- Fresh cilantro for garnish
- 6 to 7 cups mashed Yukon Gold potatoes (some varieties of white potatoes have less starch and are better for boiling). Use almond milk and a vegan butter stick when mashing.

Directions:

Heat veggie crumbles in a skillet, adding chopped onions, fresh garlic, salt, and a dash of chili powder. Sauté until onions are soft.

Prepare mashed yams and mashed potatoes, adding salt as needed.

Heat frozen vegetables.

Sauté spinach with a little olive oil until wilted.

Layer all ingredients in a 10.5 x 14.75 pan beginning with the veggie crumbles and ending with mashed russet potatoes.

Bake at 350 degrees until heated thoroughly.

To prepare cashew gravy, blend cashews and water (that they soaked in) until smooth. Heat the gravy and season with salt, pepper, and a dash of cayenne. Serve gravy over the Shepherd's pie and garnish with fresh cilantro.

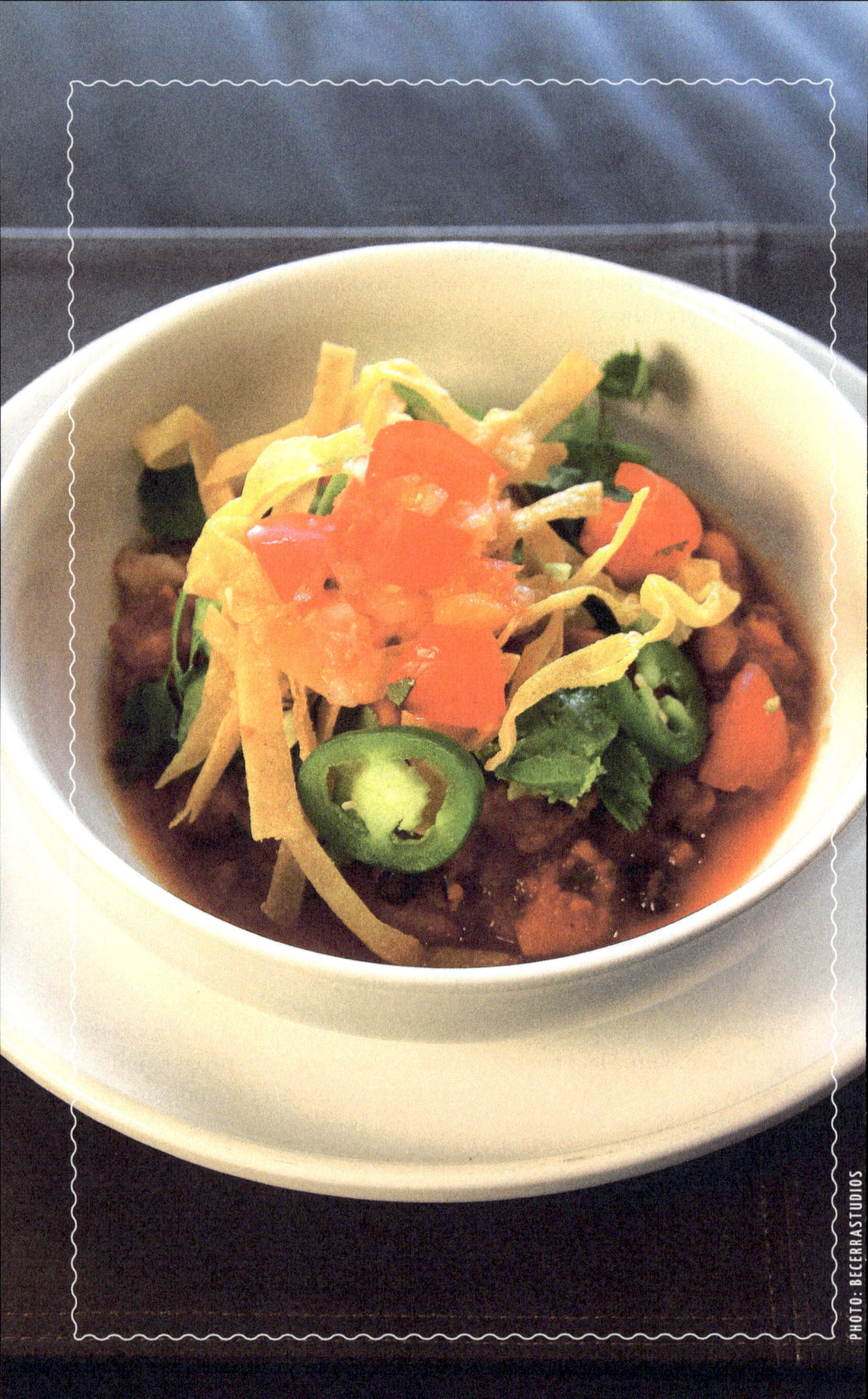

PHOTO: BECERRASTUDIOS

TEX-MEX VEGAN CHILI

Chili ingredients:

- 1 16 oz. jar organic tomato sauce
- 1 16 oz. can organic fire-roasted chopped tomatoes
- 1 small can chopped green chilies, or 1 diced Anaheim chili
- 2 cups precooked organic black beans
- 4 to 5 cups bite-sized sweet potato chunks (boiled until slightly soft and drained)
- 2-3 tbsp. chili powder (according to taste)
- 1/2 tsp. fresh chopped garlic or garlic powder
- 1/2 tsp. cayenne
- Organic pink Himalayan sea salt to taste
- 1/2 - 1 tsp. dried and ground jalapeno (use a dehydrator and prepare ahead of time for extra spicy chili)

Toppings:

- Sliced avocados
- Thinly sliced jalapenos
- 1 quartered lime
- 1 small, diced onion or fresh Pico de Gallo
- Thinly sliced, organic, yellow corn tortillas
- Fresh cilantro

Directions:

Place cooked sweet potatoes on cooking sheet and toss in olive oil and sea salt. Bake at 350 degrees for 10 minutes, or until slightly crispy. Mix all ingredients for chili together in a medium to large pot, and heat. Prepare toppings, cooking tortilla strips in hot organic canola oil until crispy then drain.

Serve chili in a bowl using the toppings of your choice!

COMPILED BY **HEATHER EDEN**

Andrea Lambert

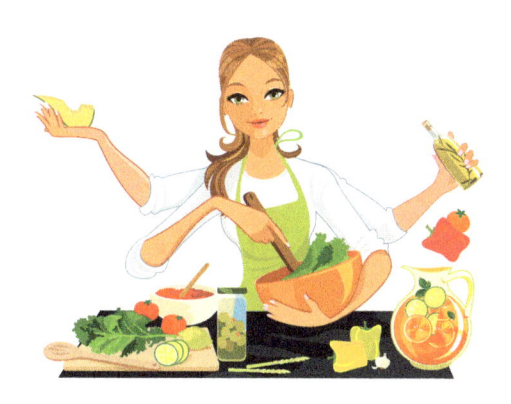

Andrea Lambert is one of Arizona's preeminent health educators and live-plant-based lifestyle experts. Since 2007, she's been focused in the studies of and participating in alternative health practices, plant-based nutrition, and endurance athletics. Andrea recently authored her first book entitled, *Life without Cancer: How to Stop Making Disease in Your Body*. She's been featured on The Food Channel, The Examiner, AZ Life and Style, and Plant Based Nation. Andrea currently teaches and coaches at An Oasis of Healing alternative cancer treatment center and maintains a successful private practice as a health educator, coach, and public speaker, empowering people to take their health into their own hands through evidence-based education!

- www.syncrawnicity.com
- www.facebook.com/syncrawnize
- www.pinterest.com/syncrawnicity

PRACTICE 20

Reflection: How Did That Meal Affect Me?

By Andrea Lambert

I first came across my current eating style after suffering pain for many years with no successful solutions from doctors. I began eating live plant-based foods (meaning uncooked fruits, veggies, nuts, seeds, and grains) after reading about their superior nutrient content, and that made sense to help my body heal. It only took thirty days to get off the dozen prescription medications I was taking for severe pain, muscle spasms, and inflammation. What I have learned over the last seven years is that this style of eating will offer the tools for anyone and everyone to heal. Additionally, this is the way to prevent illness. Following the laws of nature is our key to coming into alignment with the healthy effects of eating the way nature intended us to eat.

Becoming aware of what passes your lips can be a challenge. Number one, our culture goes too fast. Secondly, we are taught to consider food as a simple "calories in, calories out" scenario versus eating for fuel and building blocks. Lastly, we haven't been trained to pay attention to anything other than someone else or the television while we eat, and this takes our attention away from where it should be—on the proper ingestion and assimilation of the nutrients that will become our new body and energy to do the things we desire in our lives.

Eating foods that have not been thermally destroyed by heat is a primary consideration. Heat destroys nutrients and the life of the food. If we want to have high energy, we need to put food in our bodies that has high energy. For example, cooking food over 118 degrees will denature the enzymes that provide the catalyst for every chemical reaction that happens in your body. We are born with a limited supply of these enzymes. When we eat cooked foods, we require that our bodies draw on that limited, which has the effect of weakening our immune system. Additionally, chewing at a leisurely pace allows for substances like insulin to release at a slower pace, minimizing overall insulin release and maximizing blood sugar control.

Do you find yourself digging things out of the refrigerator, slapping together something "fast," and then standing at the counter to wolf it down? Do you do this while juggling the kids into their high chairs or to the kitchen table? Your kids watch and repeat what you do. Awareness is essential when we raise our kids so they have healthy role models to follow. And they will follow what you do, not what you say. Eating in a standing position with speed behind it has a negative effect on the human body.

Digestion is an activity that is governed by the parasympathetic nervous system and requires us to "rest and digest" for food to be processed efficiently. In our "hurry up and go faster" society, we need to consider how much is on our plate, figuratively and literally. Reflect on how much time you spend eating each day. The average American spends less than ten minutes consuming their lunch. It takes fifteen minutes for the first signals to be sent to the brain to let you know you're satiated. Consider that digestion starts in the mouth with chewing. Our stomachs do not have teeth, so if you don't chew well enough to begin digesting the carbohydrates with the digestive enzymes in the saliva of your mouth, it won't get chewed up and made more available for extracting nutrients in the stomach or beyond. Rushing can lead to overeating and not chewing well enough, which can lead to undigested food.

True building blocks and fuel come in the form of whole, uncooked, unadulterated fruits, veggies, nuts, seeds, and grains. This is what we were designed for and it will provide the proper calories and macro and micronutrients in the form that our bodies recognize. If we consider how much energy is in the food we are about to eat, as well as how superior or inferior the building blocks will be, our food choices will change dramatically from the Standard American Fair.

Take some time to sit with the kids, chewing completely, breathing, and teaching them to do the same instead of rushing them to the table while you eat standing, getting them to hurry up and eat before you have to rush to drop them off at school. When we take time to plan and make space for the important health aspects of our lives that keep us able to multitask, the chaos can settle a bit and we will feel the results.

Consider eating smaller portions more frequently as a time, as well. We don't have to follow all the rules society tells us to. I personally prefer to dip several sticks of celery into a pate and call it a meal. Done—lickety-split. Another meal might be a green apple dipped in raw almond butter. I will also have, at any time of the day I desire, a quick smoothie like the Simple Strawberry Smoothie. The importance of "paying attention" to your food, your body, and the effects your food has on your body is quite astounding once you begin the experiment.

Now it's time for an experiment. I'd like you to try making three simple recipes for the next twenty-one days (that's the amount of time it takes to feel the effects and change a habit). The first recipe will replace any kind of animal milk that you may have in your home. Cow's milk is the most common. I'll have you make milk out of almonds instead. The second recipe will replace breakfast and/or a snack. This will be a simple green smoothie. The last recipe will replace any kind of animal flesh (like tuna salad or chicken breast) that you might chop up and put on your salad. It's called a "pate" that you can put on your salad, dip veggies into, or even dehydrate into portable patties to eat when you only have time to sit down for a snack-sized meal.

The reason I have chosen these recipes is that they are very quick and simple to make. They taste great and can easily be adjusted to make them unique to your tastes. Replacing cow's milk is critical in the chemical age that we live in, as it contains more than double the amount of casein that's in human breast milk. This is a clue from nature showing us that we should not drink the breast milk of another species. Casein has definitively been found to be carcinogenic, and the countries that consume the most have the highest rates of osteoporosis. Once a baby has been weaned, their little bodies stop making the rennet to digest casein properly, so there is no more need for this type of food choice. When we cut dairy out of our diets, mucus production decreases in the body dramatically! Try the experiment!

The Simple Strawberry Smoothie is a great base recipe to start you off on tasty green smoothies. Try adding a banana or replacing the strawberries with blueberries. Or try adding some raw cacao powder (raw chocolate powder) with some stevia (low glycemic plant-based sweetener). You may even want to venture into some new territory and try Maca root powder to help balance your hormones and energy levels.

I chose to include a pate to offer an experience with replacing any animal flesh you might feel the need to consume. The majority of animal flesh, in America, is 60 percent fat. It is actually the fat we crave when we think we need "meat."

ALMOND MILK

Ingredients:

- 1 cup almonds (soak overnight to release enzyme inhibitors, and rinse)
- 3 cups purified water

Directions:

Blend soaked almonds and 2 cups water until smooth.

Pour through a nut milk bag or layered cheesecloth into a pitcher and squeeze the liquid, leaving the pulp behind. Freeze the pulp for later recipes, like raw cakes.

The milk will last about 3 to 4 days refrigerated. Optional adds: stevia or dates, vanilla or cinnamon. Try a variety of raw nuts like Brazil, hazelnut, and pistachio.

SIMPLE STRAWBERRY SMOOTHIE

Ingredients:

- 1/4 cup almonds
- 1 large handful of spinach
- 1 cup strawberries
- Purified water, as needed

Directions:

Blend almonds with 1 cup of water until smooth.

Add spinach and strawberries, blending until smooth.

Give it a taste and try adding a bit a stevia and Himalayan salt and adjust it to your taste.

Drink right away or sip over several hours, but do not store due to oxidation of nutrients (an apple browns, losing it nutrients when it's cut).

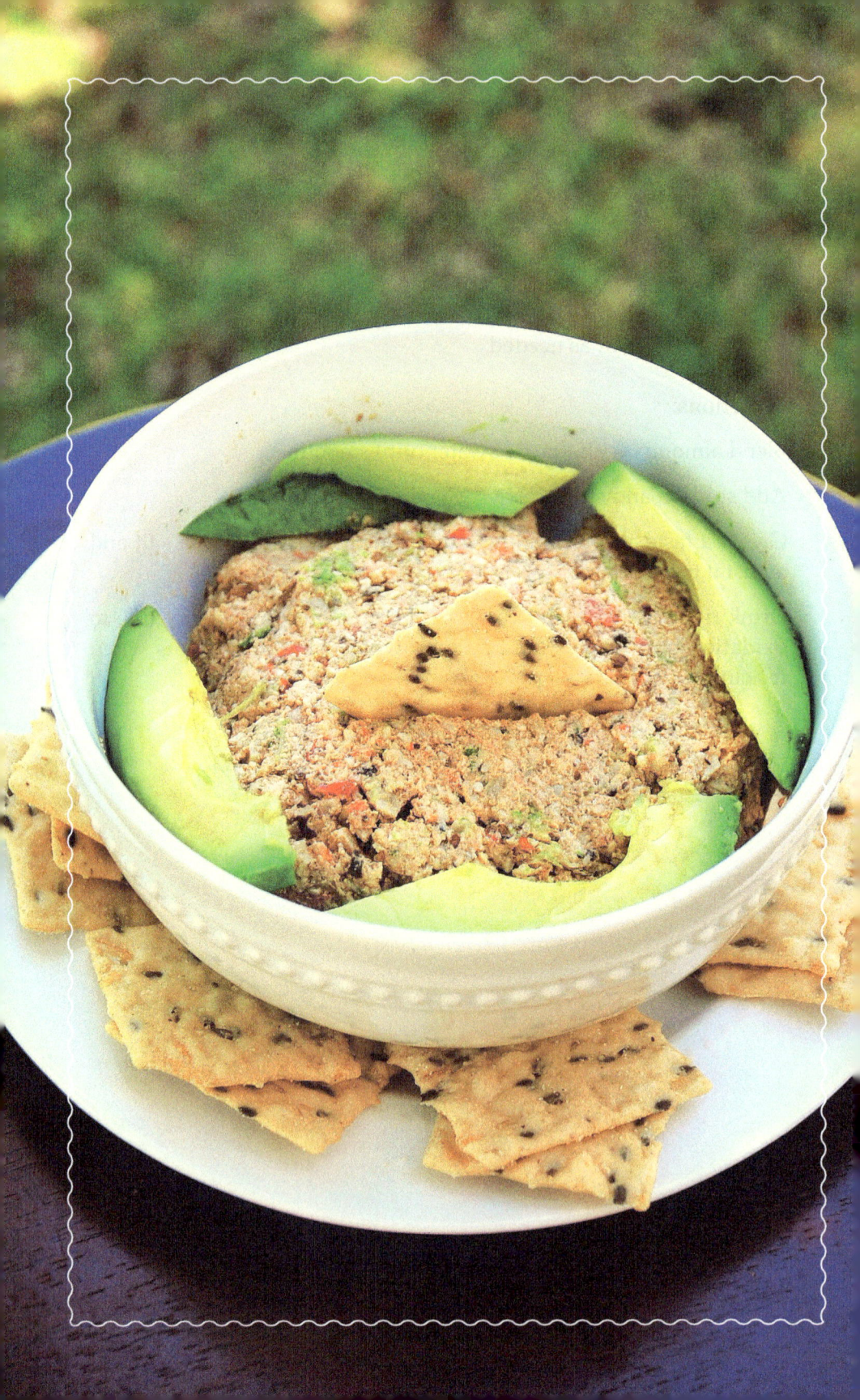

WINNING WALNUT PATE

Ingredients:

- 2 cups walnuts
- 2 ribs celery
- 2 scallions
- 1 red bell pepper
- 1 tsp. Celtic salt

Directions:

Blend all ingredients in food processor until smooth.

Will keep refrigerated for about a week.

BALANCE FOR **BUSY MOMS**

COMPILED BY **HEATHER EDEN**

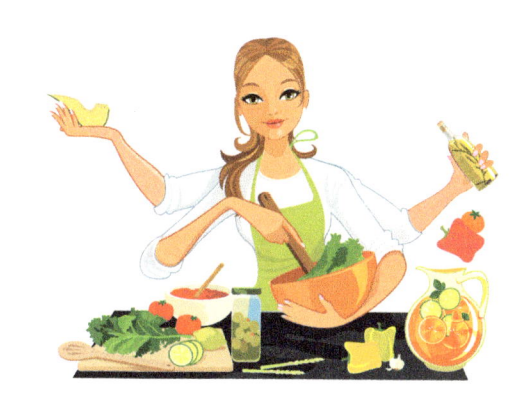

Sally Eisenberg, CHC, AADP

Sally is a health coach certified by the Institute for Integrative Nutrition and Columbia University and accredited by the Association of Drugless Practitioners. She holds a BS in marketing from Drexel University and is the founder of Nourish Ur Life, a nutrition/healthy lifestyle practice located in Philadelphia, PA. As a mom and multimedia artist, Sally has always been passionate about food and healthy living and integrating nutritional counseling with her artistic vision. In addition to working with private clients, Sally offers cooking classes out of her home, empowering her attendees to cook healthfully in their OWN kitchens.

- www.nourishurlife.com
- sally@nourishurlife.com
- www.facebook.com/NourishUrLife
- www.twitter.com/NourishUrLife
- www.instagram.com/nourishlife.com
- www.nourishurlife.blogspot.com
- www.linkedin.com/in/sallyeisenberg

PRACTICE 21

Exploring the Senses

By Sally Eisenberg, CHC, AADP

We generally associate eating with our sense of taste. But the act of cooking and consuming food is a decidedly multisensory experience. As we chop, sauté, and chew, we engage all of our senses: sight, smell, touch, and sound, along with taste. Harnessing these sensory experiences during the cooking and preparation process heightens enjoyment while encouraging us to pay attention to the act of eating. When we fully engage with our food, great things will happen in the mind AND body:

- We experience a more wholesome and enjoyable eating experience;
- We enhance digestion; and,
- We maintain our optimum, healthy weight.

With our busy, hectic lives, it becomes increasingly easy to get caught up in the "grab and go" style of eating—a quick fix to put something into our bodies. Instead of deliberately considering the important act of eating, we feel constantly rushed and unsatisfied, causing our stomachs to fight back with indigestion and discomfort. Consuming food in a hurried, frenetic way precludes us from listening to our bodies and paying attention to what positively or negatively impacts our digestion. Everyone's body is different, with varied food needs and intolerances. When we allow ourselves the time to enjoy the act of eating, we experience a lifestyle filled with ease rather than disease.

It may sound strange, but it takes work to truly connect with our bodies and digestive systems. For example, in times of stress, we often turn to "comfort" foods to compensate for the anxiety we're experiencing.

We think these dishes, which are often over-indulgent and unhealthy, will make us feel better and mitigate the stress. However, they do just the opposite. As we gorge on "comfort" foods we end up feeling extremely *un*comfortable!

Consider my own experience: During my teenage and early adult years, I frequently turned to unhealthy foods when experiencing tension or stress. I would raid my junk food collection with fervor, thinking nothing of going for all of them at once. I would first eat something sweet, then switch to salty, and then back again. This would continue until I wrought havoc on both my stomach and brain, and craved a piece of celery to stabilize my bingeing. Food yoyo-ing, rapid consumption, and unhealthy bingeing gave me no satisfaction, when in fact I was looking for comfort *from* eating. I could have avoided the feeling of discomfort, bloating, and disdain at my over-eating if I had approached my food with my senses.

Eating with our senses is ingrained in humans from birth. As we age, and become caught up in our fast-paced existences, we unlearn the delight of the eating experience. Observing a young child in the act of eating reminds us of the essential nature of sensory consumption. I remember feeding my daughter solids for the first time. She loved sweet potatoes. She would listen as I spooned the sweet potatoes on to her plate, looking at the starchy orange vegetable with total delight. Then, with her tiny fingers, she would mush the potato, before bringing a bite to her lips to taste. She totally immersed herself in the sweet potatoes, while I thrilled in the presence of her beautiful experience of mindful eating.

We can learn so much from our children's first experiences with food. Unlike many of us, they aren't multi-tasking by reading the newspaper, catching up on e-mails, or texting. They aren't watering the plants or wiping the counter while fitting in a bite here and there. They are simply enjoying their food in the most primal way; paying attention to each mouthful and to their parent who strives to keep them safe, happy, and well-fed.

Here are some recommendations I give to my clients as I guide them in exploring all of their senses around food. Try practicing these with your kids, as well. It is a fun way to engage with them around food:

- As you get ready to eat ANYTHING, make sure you sit down with your food and nothing else (keep your devices in another room).
- Take a deep breath as soon as you sit down in front of your plate.
- Think about how grateful you are for the food you are about to eat.
- Begin to engage your senses...
- Engage the sense of sight. What does the food look like? What colors are present? Is it flat? Round? Layered? Sharp? Soft?
- Engage the sense of smell. Does the food smell sweet? Fresh? Strong? Mild? Floral? Bitter?
- Engage the sense of touch. Does it feel smooth? Is it grainy? Is it soft? Is it gritty? Tender? Flaky? Mushy? Dry? Wet?
- Engage the sense of sound. What do you hear when you take a bite? Does the bite make a crunchy sound? A swish? A slurp?
- Engage your sense of taste. Does the food taste sweet? Savory? Spicy? Sour? Bitter? Bland?
- Focus on chewing each bite. The more time you take with each bite, the more you will break down the food by releasing digestive enzymes, allowing you to easily absorb the nutrients fully into your body, reducing indigestion and creating less gas. In addition, the more you focus on chewing, the more full you will become and the less food you will consume. Your body will thank you!

We are role models to our kids when it comes to food and mindfulness. As they grow older, they have their own distractions. Practicing these recommendations will bring you (and your children) to a more mindful state of eating, which will have many positive effects—both physical *and* mental. Remember, eating with our senses is a practice that will become easier and more comfortable with time.

I invite you and your kids to experiment with the two recipes in this chapter. They are simple, tasty, and will invigorate all of your senses!

SALLY'S RAW ZUCCHINI PASTA WITH PEPPERS, AVOCADO, AND APPLE CIDER VINEGAR

Yield: 2 Servings

Ingredients: (organic if possible)

- 1 medium to large zucchini
- 1/2 red pepper, diced
- 1/2 orange pepper, diced
- 1 avocado, diced
- 1/8 cup raw apple cider vinegar
- 1/4 cup extra virgin olive oil
- 1/4 tsp. oregano
- Sea salt and pepper, to taste
- Fresh parsley (for garnish)

Directions:

If you want the zucchini to look more like authentic spaghetti, peel before slicing. Because the skin offers an excellent source of fiber to the dish, I prefer not to peel. The skin also enhances the dish with a brilliant pop of color.

Slice the zucchini vertically in very thin strips. If you have a spiralizer, the tool will do it for you, and it's so much fun to use with (or without) the kids. I use the Paderno World Cuisine brand, available at Amazon. Once sliced, place the zucchini strips in a bowl and add in the diced peppers.

In a separate bowl, whisk together all of the other ingredients, except for the avocado. When finished, pour over the zucchini, mix together, and top with the diced avocado and fresh parsley.

Enjoy!

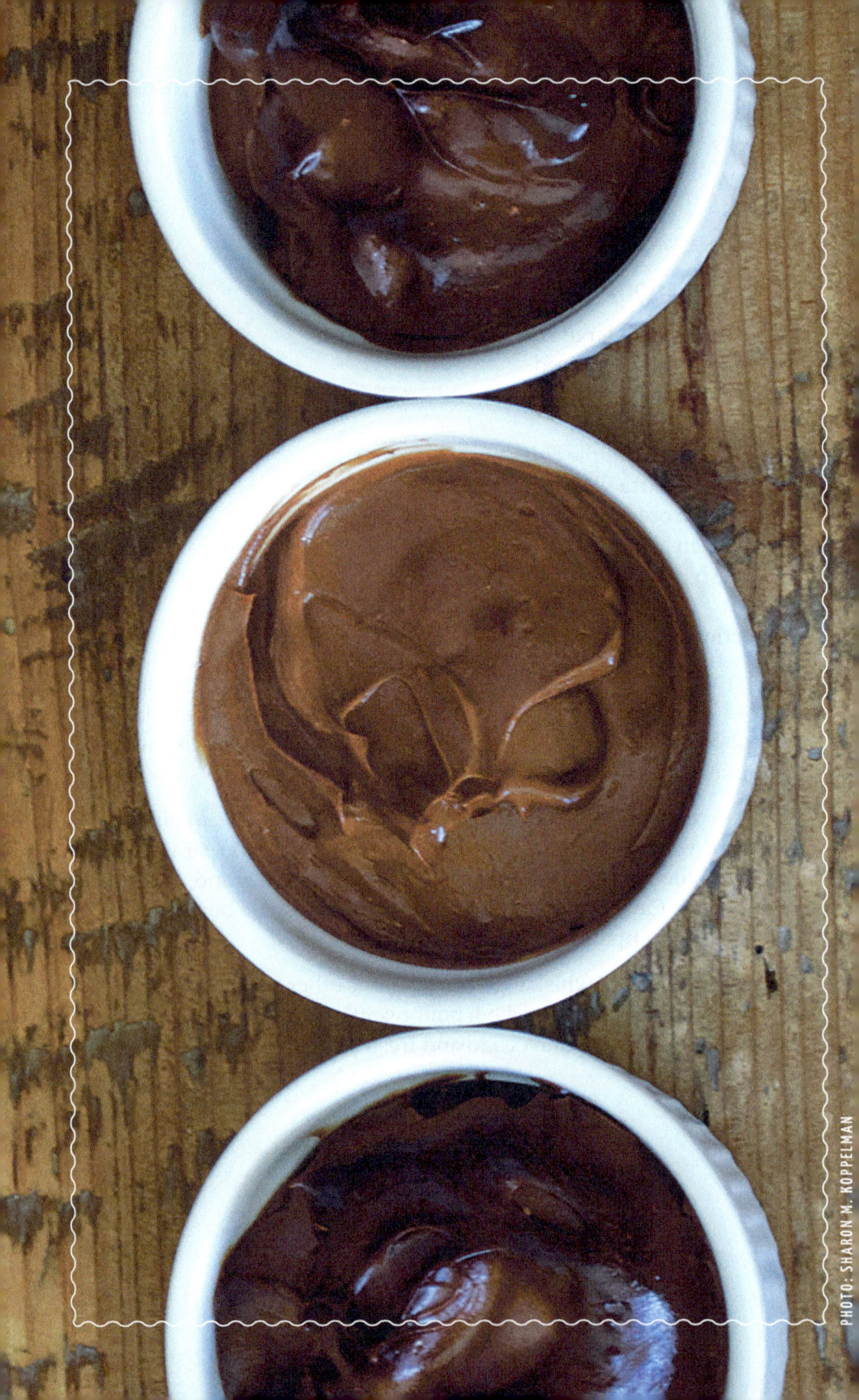

PHOTO: SHARON M. KOPPELMAN

RAW CHOCOLATE SEA SALT PUDDING

Yield: 6 servings

Chocolate pudding continues to be one of my all-time favorite desserts. This recipe will not only satisfy your chocolate cravings but will offer nutritional benefits for the entire family, including healthy fats, vitamins, minerals, and antioxidants.

Ingredients:

- 3 avocados, peeled from skin and pits removed
- 6 tbsp. raw cacao powder
- 1/2 cup pure maple syrup
- 1 tsp. pure vanilla extract
- 1/4 cup filtered water
- Pinch sea salt

Directions:

Blend in a high-speed blender until smooth. Use more or less water, depending on your desired consistency. Spoon the pudding into small ramekins. Place in refrigerator to chill. When ready to serve, sprinkle with a pinch of coarse sea salt and be ready to wow everyone in your household. Chocolate pudding never tasted so good!

COMPILED BY **HEATHER EDEN**

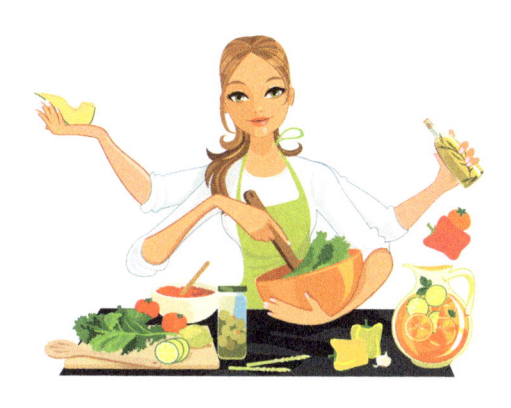

Patti Hedrick, CHHC, AADP

Patti Hedrick is the founder of Love Nourish Live. She is a board certified Holistic Health and Lifestyle Coach and a member of American Association of Drugless Practitioners (AADP). She received her certification from the Institute of Integrative Nutrition and continued her education with a more intense functional nutrition training where she earned her Holistic Nutrition Lab Full Body Systems Certification. Patti specializes in getting clients to improve their food choices and have an overall increase in happiness with their lives. She integrates a holistic approach by taking into account all areas of their lives and supplying the necessary tools for lifelong changes.

- ✉ patti@lovenourishlive.com
- 🏠 www.lovenourishlive.com
- f www.facebook.com/pages/Love-Nourish-Live/117418048352394?ref=hl
- ⓟ www.pinterest.com/lovenourishlive/

PRACTICE 22

Degrees of Awareness

By Patti Hedrick, CHHC, AADP

I am going to write this as though you are sitting in front of me, and you are one of my clients. Let's both start by taking a long, slow deep breath in; and now release it slowly. So, let's talk about degrees of awareness. Awareness to me is when you are conscious of something. There are degrees of awareness in every part of our life, from relationships to food choices!

I like to break it down into three levels: Good, Better, and Best. I noticed as a mom, I was making the best choices for my son—by making his organic baby food, breast feeding, etc.—but never for me. After I weaned my son from breastfeeding, I started my "three pots a day of coffee and sugar" diet plan. I was a complete mess. Sure, I was moving and grooving and getting things done, but I was a mess. This new diet plan had me going nowhere fast, and I ended up chubby, moody, and tired. It added a new thing in my life called anxiety. I told my doctor, "Not me, it has to be something else." First thing I did was eliminate the caffeine.

My doctor wanted me to take meds, and if you knew me, you'd know I never could do that. I am not saying it is wrong, but I wanted to do this the all-natural way. So my doctor introduced me to guided meditation on the Internet. From there, it just led me to other holistic things. I started to become more mindful of what I was doing and how I was doing it. Then I started going to an acupuncturist. I felt better after the first session. My acupuncturist was helping with my different degrees of awareness, but it was more on the level of doing too much—you know multitasking without asking for help. He made me promise to do just one thing and enjoy it, even if it was doing the dishes. I just laughed, but promised I would apply it to my day. The old me wanted to cook, run around the house, and play the pickup game before my husband returned home. I stuck to my promise and just cooked. I did not burn a thing. That very "chore" I used to love and then hated? I found love for again. I played music and really just enjoyed myself cooking. Yes, one thing at a time. Oh, the joy. You will find this joy again. Just start to flex that mindfulness muscle again.

Let's get back to you! Do you rush to get a dinner on the table and not sit down at all? Inevitably, somebody will need something that is amazingly NOT on the table. So your dinner ends up cold, or you're eating scraps over the sink. First thing I want you to do is make yourself AWARE of your eating habits. Are you sitting down to a home-cooked meal? Are you grateful and giving time for prayer before you eat? Do you take your time and chew your food and eat with a certain level of awareness?

My "good, better, best" theory is what I share with my clients. I was there making the same unaware choices most moms do when they have so many other things on their to-do list. Takeout seems easier and faster, or some processed thing in a box that you just microwave seems to work better. When you do go grocery shopping, use my "good, better, best" theory.

Let me give you an example. I would love a plateful of French fries. They are easy to make, kids love them, and I am craving them.

PATTI'S "GOOD, BETTER, BEST" THEORY:

Good: Buy a bag of frozen French fries and bake them in the oven. They are not deep fried and I control the salt!

Better: Buy a bag of organic, non-GMO French fries and bake them.

Best: Buy organic sweet potatoes, cut them up, and put amazing seasonings on them—like turmeric, cumin, cinnamon, sea salt, etc., and bake them.

Different degrees of awareness, wouldn't you say? My theory will bring about awareness to all of the choices you are making for you and your family.

Now let's talk about mindless eating. Bring awareness into the picture. Be conscious of what you are snacking on at 7:00 p.m., when the children are sleeping and you feel relaxed. Why are you eating? Are you hungry, bored, upset with someone? The awareness here happens when you realize that your mind has control over your body. This is where you can really make some great changes. Be mindful of what you are putting in your body. We must become so in tune with our bodies that we can actually feel the food energy from what we are consuming. Are you nourishing your body? Somewhere in your degree of awareness, there has to be an awaking in your spirit. This is a never-ending itch to be scratched, so to speak. You will always be working at some level in every area of your life on different degrees of awareness. So always work towards the BEST choice for your body.

Here are some simple steps to follow: Ask yourself if you are hungry. If you are, what degree of awareness are you going to apply here? It should be the BEST level for food choices after 7:00 p.m., because anything after is going to be hard on your digestive tract. Your body needs time to digest and overall, it just makes you healthier.

Another factor that will just happen when you are more aware is you will start to cook more in your kitchen. You will start to play around with healthier ingredients and different recipes with "good, better, best" foods! You will start to eat more at home and less out because you are becoming more aware of how really horrible takeout is. Getting back into the kitchen for me was a spiritual process and everything I do, I do with love and excitement. The end result is everyone is always happy and you are nourishing you and your family with whole foods you made. It takes all those guessing games out of your mind. All of this is eliminated because the chef is you!

In the last part of our session, I want you to be aware of what is actually in your food. Read the labels. Does an apple have an ingredient label? This is why whole foods are so much better for you. Your body recognizes this type of food and knows how to use it. This food has life-force energy. Pick up a box or bag of anything and try reading what is in it. My rule of thumb is, if you do not know what an ingredient is, don't eat it. A really easy way is if it has more than five ingredients in it, don't buy it. Be careful of the food label claims on the outside of the package. Start to raise your awareness of things you are buying.

I really enjoyed this session with you. Remember: always work toward a certain degree of awareness in every area of your life. This brings on excitement and healthy changes. You won't believe how things in your life start to align themselves!

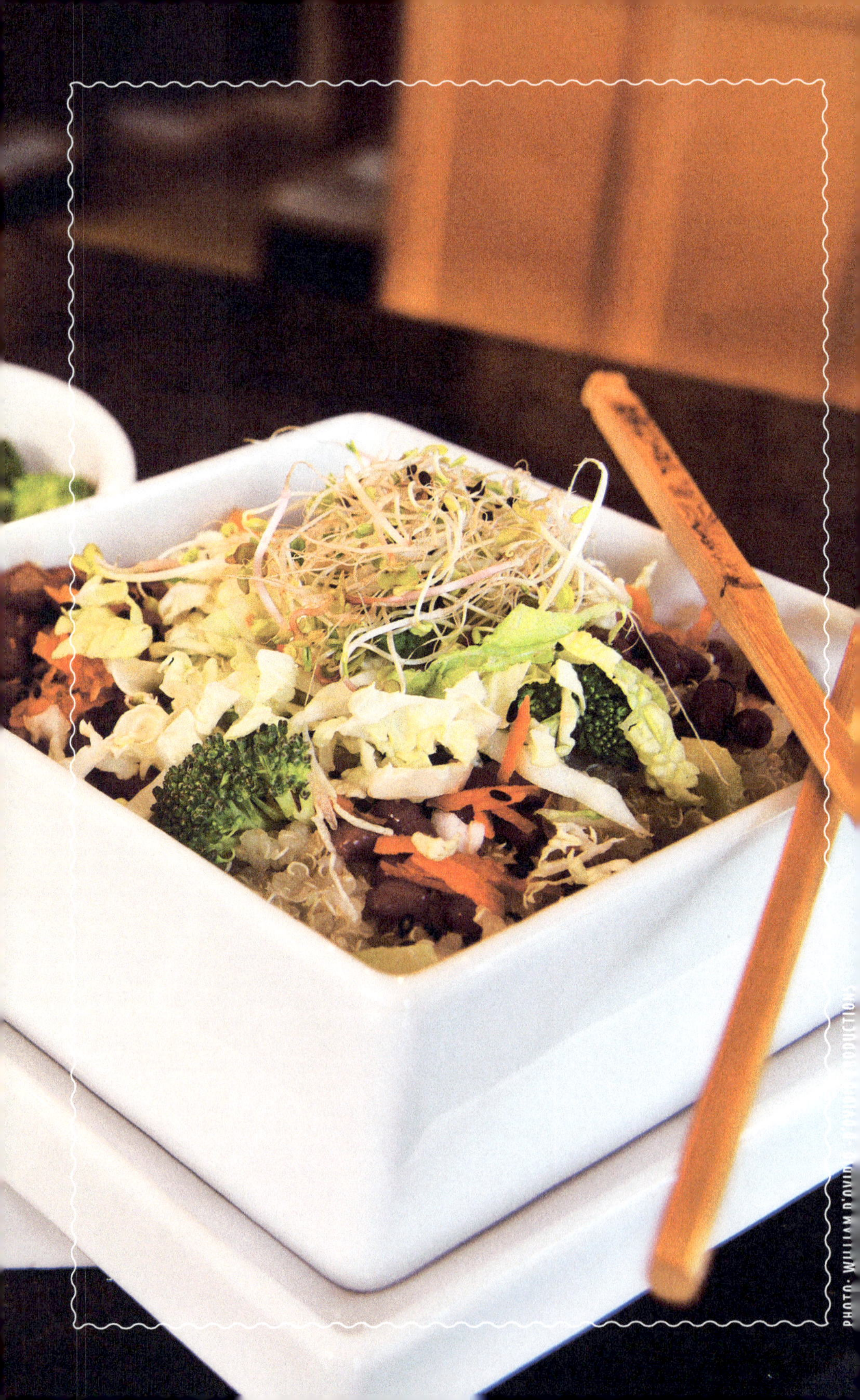

PHOTO: WILLIAM D'OVID[illegible]ODUCTIONS

ASIAN BUDDHA BOWL

Servings: 2

Ingredients:

- 2 cups cooked quinoa, brown rice, or rice noodles
- Adzuki beans or any protein (fish, chicken)
- 2 shredded carrots
- 1 cup broccoli
- 1 diced green onion
- 1 garlic clove minced
- Raw greens and sprouts

Directions:

Cook quinoa. Cut all veggies into small bite-size pieces. Cook protein of your choice. I just sauté the beans for a little bit in some olive oil and added the garlic and onions. You may also add broccoli and carrots, if you like them to be warm. Place quinoa in two separate bowls then place beans and vegetables. Add greens and sprouts and cover with sauce.

Easy Sauce:

- 4 tbsp. low sodium tamari Sauce
- 1 tsp. of honey or maple syrup

ZUCCHINI FRIES

Ingredients:

- 3 zucchinis
- 1 cup panko crumbs
- 1 tbsp. organic Italian seasoning
- Sea salt
- 1/4 cup shredded parmesan cheese
- 2 organic eggs

Directions:

Preheat oven to 425 degrees. Line a cookie sheet with parchment paper and lightly spray with oil. Cut your zucchini. Lightly sprinkle with salt. Combine panko crumbs, organic Italian seasoning, and shredded parmesan cheese in a shallow dish. Whisk eggs together and dip each zucchini fries into the egg, coating well in panko mixture. Set on the cookie sheet. Bake for 15 to 20 minutes, until lightly brown. Fries can be flipped halfway through baking time.

Dipping sauce:

Easy: Buy any organic marinara sauce. Heat on stovetop and sprinkle with parmesan cheese.

Fun: 1/4 cup Greek yogurt, 1 tbsp. organic mayo, Sriracha to your liking, dash of salt

COMPILED BY **HEATHER EDEN**

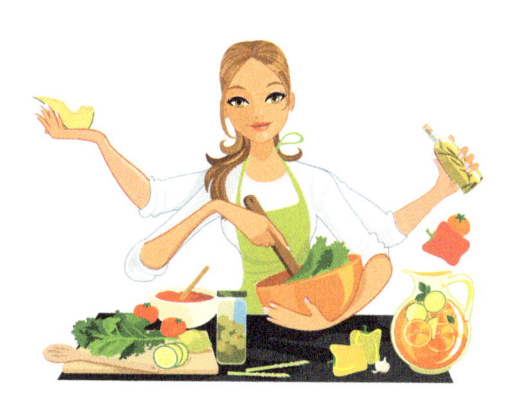

Marika Tomkins

Marika is a wellness warrior who empowers maxed-out mamas and spent professionals to recreate their health and lifestyle. She is the founder and owner Your Best Health and Self, a certified brown belt Nia instructor, and doTerra wellness advocate. Marika provides a loving, intuitive, and wisdom-rich environment for her clients to incorporate a nutrient-rich diet, detox, personal care, and to pursue their dreams. Her signature offerings include seasonal Glow detoxes, the three-month Body, Mind, Spirit Make Over, and the six-month Empowered Wellness for Warriors. Marika received her BA from Whitman College and her CHHC from the Institute for Integrative Nutrition.

See link below to get your own pdf of Your Unique Experience map.

- marika@marikatomkins.com
- healthcoach.marika
- www.marikatomkins.com
- www.nianow.com/marikatomkins
- marikatomkins.com/youruniqueexperience
- www.facebook.com/marikatomkinshealthcoach
- 509.876.1109

Walla Walla, WA

PRACTICE 23

Your Unique Experience

By Marika Tomkins

As a busy mom, business owner, wellness instructor, and follower of dreams, I deeply understand how food can be the cornerstone of feeling empowered in multiple arenas, as well as how it can sabotage great intentions and unravel confidence and self-esteem. Through many years of wellness training and coursework at the Institute for Integrative Nutrition, I have come to understand the importance of personal truth telling and taking ownership of my own unique experience with food. I invite you to grab a cup of tea, a journal, and come along with me for some self-discovery to create a personal pathway for peace and freedom with food.

Are you ready to have food create more energy, a stronger immune system, glowing self-esteem, healthy weight, self-love, and beauty? I have learned in order to have great practices with food that yield results, most of us need to roll up our sleeves and get honest with ourselves about how and why we relate the way we do with food. My own unique experience with food is that, while I am an aficionado of whole foods, greens prepared 101 ways, traditional food practices, superfoods, and kitchen gadgets, my truth is I relate to my food as an emotional eater who will binge when my gut, my life, or my nervous system is out of balance.

Shifting my relationship with food meant taking *ownership* of my own unique experience with food—*my story*. Seeing myself clearly empowered me to truly prioritize overall balance and sense when my life, schedule, and gut need extra care.

Are you ready? Let's dive in together and look at your unique experience—*your truth*. Identifying your own experience with food and nutrition will make it easier for you to acknowledge what's working, what isn't, and some simple steps that will make you feel like the amazing woman and mama you are.

1. Map your food experience. What has food been like at each stage of your life? What have been your most healthy and balanced experiences with food? What have been your least healthy? Take ten minutes and write your own eating story, starting as a child. What trends do you notice?

My map of positive food connections includes: fascination with healthy recipes, a love of sharing and preparing foods for others, learning from other people and cultures. The not helpful practices: getting too hungry, putting too much performance pressure on myself and schedule, feeling overwhelmed with difficult emotions such as fear and loneliness.

2. Map your practical day-to-day beneficial practices and wellness blocker behaviors. Make a chart with a line down the middle and write down at least twenty things that work and twenty more things that do not work. Be specific.

My beneficial practices:

1. Sharing and preparing food with others.

2. Eating out of my own garden.

3. Detoxing with each of the four seasons.

4. The art of baking with natural sugars and non-gluten grains or grain-free.

5. Doing an elimination diet.

6. Journaling and mediation.

7. Regular exercise and self-expression.

8. Using essential oils topically, aromatically, and internally.

9. Packing my lunch with dinner leftovers.

10. Being honest with myself and friendships that enable me to explore my truth.

WHAT DOESN'T WORK?

Easy access to homemade baked goods in my home or office.

Skipping meals.

Going to the office without healthy food.

Upholding strict diets that make me feel deprived.

Eating when in privacy because no one is looking.

Serving myself too small of a portion and then refilling my plate.

Processed wheat, dairy, and corn.

Too full of a schedule and unrealistic expectations.

Expensive hot, sugary drinks.

Negative self-talk.

3. Be honest. Now that you have mapped what food habits propel you into feeling great and taking good care of yourself and noticed what food behaviors send you into feeling crappy and out of balance, it is time to declare your truth. What is it?

My truth: Due to my history of being an emotional eater and binger, I must take extra care of my wellbeing to safeguard my healthy relationship with food. When I notice myself engaging in food habits that don't work, I know it is time to slow down, choose a few beneficial practices, and access the love and support of a trusted friend, colleague, or coach.

4. Do an elimination diet, anywhere from seven to twenty-eight days. Elimination diets, in my opinion, are hands down the best way to determine your own unique wellness blueprint. Simply eliminate gluten, corn, soy, dairy, sugar and *all* processed foods for your specific amount of time and notice how you feel. At the end of your designated period, add one food back in every three days and see how your body responds. If you have a negative response, test it two more times to be sure. Remove any foods from your diet that elicit a sensitive response.

I personally do elimination diets during my seasonal detoxes to continually get clear about what foods serve me and what foods deplete me. It takes time and experimentation to become masterful at hearing what your body is telling you. Experience is the best teacher here.

5. Commit to a personal wellness practice. Make a practice of making time for your physical, mental, emotional, and spirit wellness. Make a long list of activities that bring you inner peace and ones that you would like to try. Identify which ones you can easily fold into your life—hint choose ones that can be done in fifteen minutes to an hour and can be done at home or out with friends. Commit, for the long haul, to incorporating your wellness practices into your life. As the expression goes, "When mama ain't happy, no one is happy."

My tools: Teaching, practicing, and taking Nia classes, meditation, photography, gardening, walking, writing, and regular time nurturing at least three friendships.

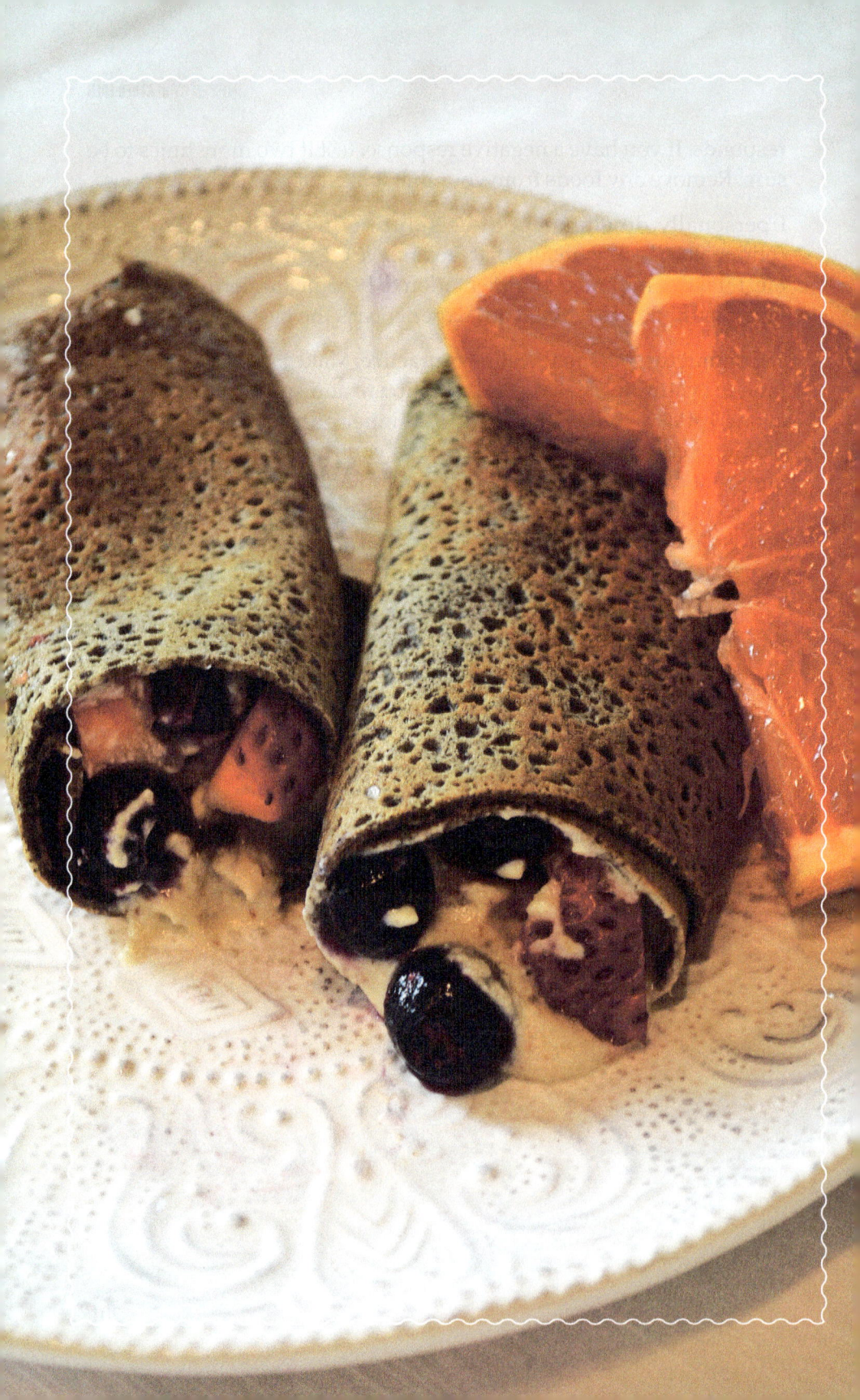

BUCKWHEAT CASHEW LOVE FILLED CREPES

Serves 4 to 8, depending on what else you are serving

FOR CREPES:

- 2 cups pasture-raised milk or nondairy almond or coconut milk
- 1 1/4 cups buckwheat flour
- 6 eggs
- 3 tbsp. coconut oil or grass-fed butter
- 1 tsp honey
- Pinch of salt

Directions:

Blend all ingredients in blender or mixer. Crepes come out better when the batter has a chance to rest. I recommend mixing the batter up the night before, or a couple of hours prior to cooking.

FOR CASHEW CRÈME:

- 1 cup cashews, soaked for a few hours or overnight, rinsed and drained
- 4 to 5 Medjool dates
- Vanilla to your preferred taste
- Cold water to cover cashews

Directions:

Blend ingredients until smooth and set aside.

FRUIT FILLING:

- 3 to 4 cups of cut-up fruit and berries

Directions:

Preheat skillet or crepe pan to medium.

Stir the crepe batter as you go, as the buckwheat tends to settle towards the bottom.

Melt a little coconut oil or butter onto pan for the first crepe.

Pour approximately 1/4 cup of the crepe batter into pan and swirl it around so that the batter thinly covers the entire surface.

Cook each side for about 20 to 30 seconds.

Assemble cashew crème and fruit into crepe, roll, and serve.

Kids and adults love this dish. Crepe batter keeps well in the fridge for up to 3 days.

BRUSSELS SPROUT POMEGRANATE CELEBRATION SALAD

Serves 4 to 6

Ingredients:

- 1 1/4 pounds Brussels sprouts, stems removed
- 1 red pear, thinly sliced
- 1 pomegranate, de-seeded*
- 1/3 cup toasted and chopped hazelnuts
- 1/2 cup olive oil
- 1/4 cup lemon juice (one large lemon)
- 1 tbsp. Dijon mustard
- 2 tbsp. raw apple cider vinegar
- 2 to 3 tbsp. honey
- Salt

Directions:

Bring 2 quarts of water to boil in large pot. Prepare Brussels sprouts by shredding with knife or sending through a food processor. Blanche Brussels sprouts in boiling water and drain in colander. Cool immediately with cold water. Place colander aside and allow water to drain. Pat dry with towel.

In large bowl, whisk together olive oil and Dijon. Slowly whisk in lemon juice and vinegar, creating an emulsion. Stir in honey and salt to taste. Pour dressing into jar.

Toss Brussels sprouts into bowl and add dressing. Reserve any leftover dressing. Mix in pomegranate seeds. Garnish with pear slices and hazelnuts on each plate, or present in bowl. Serve immediately.

Tip: Make salad ahead and place in fridge. Garnish with pears and hazelnuts just before serving.

Tip for de-seeding pomegranate: Cut ends of pomegranate and cut skin into quarters from top to bottom. Break fruit apart and place in water. This part is messy, so be prepared with an apron and a towel to wipe the mess. Free the seeds from pomegranate skin and membranes in water. The seeds will sink to the bottom and the membrane and thick outside skin will float to the top.

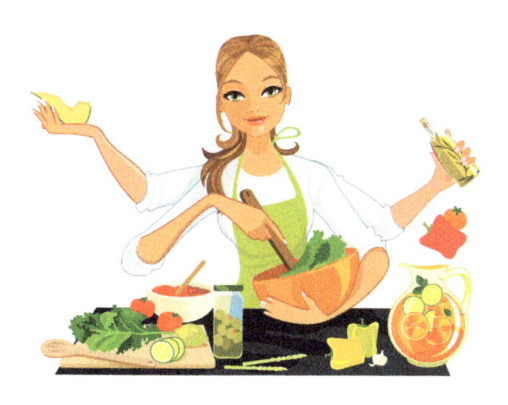

Jacqueline Allen

Jacqueline created Dynamic Health Consulting in 2013. she's a yoga teacher, board certified holistic health practitioner, and member of the American Association of Drugless Practitioners. In 2001, she created The Pathwork to Conscious Living, a healing arts counseling business that focuses on the concept of spirituality being maturation of the personality, hands-on healing techniques, chakra balancing and restructuring, clearing childhood wounds, working with defenses, character structures, and relationships. She's a Reiki master and minister, having performed many weddings. Living with her beloved Jack, she spends quality time with her grandchildren, enjoying the Great Northwest lifestyle, where she was born and raised.

- Jacqueline@DynamicHealthConsulting.com
- www.Dynamichealthconsulting.com (Receive a free E-book when you sign up for her newsletter.)
- www.facebook.com/dynamichealthconsulting
- www.linkedin.com/in/dynamichealthconsulting/
- www.twitter.com/dynamichealth2u/

PRACTICE 24

I Eat to Live a Healthy, Vibrant Life!

By Jacqueline Allen

I was twelve years old and old enough to ride the bus by myself to the berry fields.

I was so excited. It was my chance to earn some money. Rows upon rows of the biggest strawberries I had ever seen. Well, you can guess how it went: eat, pick, eat, pick, and eat some more. I was actually good at it—eating and picking. When strawberries were finished, I ventured to raspberries. I thought I was in heaven—such wonderful pure food, and so plentiful. I became pretty good at this picking job. At some point, I realized I needed to put some in the bin to make money.

So as I got older, I graduated to bigger and better job opportunities. I stayed in Wenatchee during the summer months with my cousins, and we all picked in the orchards. Wow! Cherries, peaches, pears—so yummy! We eventually graduated from the orchards to the packing sheds. We enjoyed shopping for clothes and summer fun activities, especially the teen dances on Saturday nights.

To this day, one of my favorite things to do with my partner Jack is to go to the U-pick farms and pick thirty gallons of raspberries, blueberries, and blackberries. We freeze them for our smoothies we drink every day. I absolutely love opening a bag of berries I know we picked. When I open a bag of blackberries and smell that fresh scent of summer, it takes me right there again, to the day I picked them, and then back to being a young girl with Mom and all my sisters, out in the woods, with a stick and pail in tow. The stick was for lifting up the sticker bushes, and there they were—beautiful wild fresh blackberries. The ones the bears eat, and yes, we all were running for our lives one summer day when we were out in the woods. I heard my aunt scream, "BEAR!!!" We ran as fast as we could for the car—over logs and through sticker bushes. We got back to the car safely but with plenty of scratches and scared for our lives. But apparently not scared enough…we just found another place to pick. Living in the Northwest, there are plenty of woods.

Being sixty-two, mom and grandparent, yoga instructor, and health coach, I know what makes my body feel good. I believe it is necessary to listen to our bodies; it will speak to us, always.

When we are tuned in, with awareness, we choose from our inner knowing. This has served me in so many ways throughout my life, in what I eat to how much I eat. Of course, I have fallen to temptation. I am just like anyone else. When I do eat something that makes me feel less than good, I suffer, so that suffering imprints on my cellular level. My next food choice is a better choice, one that makes me feel good. It is that simple—know thyself!

So I experiment with good foods. I stay away from the nightshade family because it causes inflammation in my joints and bunion on my right foot. I feel it immediately, when I eat tomatoes that are processed, peanuts, potatoes, eggplants, or peppers. My bunion will throb with pain.

I focus on superfoods, such as flax seeds, chia seeds, hemp protein powder, and blue-green algae—another great source of vegetable protein, keffir for probiotics that I make myself, and mushrooms because they are especially good for immune-building properties. There are studies that have been done that suggest that one mushroom a day will cut your chances of certain cancers by 40 percent. I blend all this together in my morning smoothie—one of our handpicked berry selections. A banana is always included, along with baby kale— another source of vegetable protein. I include cinnamon for balancing my blood sugar, and for great taste. I also include some Indian spice. I love the flavors of these spices. I grind up fennel, cardamom, cumin, and some turmeric for inflammation. Turmeric is an analgesic—an anti- inflammatory. One tsp. a day is a beneficial pain reliever, too.

Remember, "I eat to live a healthy, vibrant life…at sixty-two!" It is working! No illness and I have plenty of energy. I believe HEALTH is WEALTH. My mom died at age fifty-seven from cancer, caused by smoking and a very high-stressed life. I was determined to be a healthy person at a young age after witnessing my father's health problems and how much he was affected by his stroke at age thirty-two. The stress and lifestyle of both my parents taught me what I didn't want to be.

I maintained my lifestyle and health until my late thirties, until I needed a hysterectomy. I believed if I exercised enough I would be healthy. Stress and exposure to toxins caused hormonal disruption. It took years to get back where I needed to be. I love how the Universe has put me in the right place at the right time, leading me where I needed to be. Researching on my own, I discovered a holistic approach to health, and healed myself. I later found the Institute for Integrative Nutrition, and I am now a holistic health coach and a board certified member of the American Association of Drugless Practitioners. I can now share my knowledge and help others be the best they can be.

Eating locally is a recommended sustainable eating practice. It supports our local farmers and local fish markets and sustains our economy. Studies indicate that the healthiest food choices are within one hundred miles of your kitchen table.

You can guess that my favorite local food is berries. I have shared my healthy recipe for them in my morning smoothies. Enjoy! My partner Jack and I always grow a nice garden. There couldn't be anything more local than your own garden. We have over sixteen blueberry plants, and raspberries too. We can trust what we are eating because we grew it. We know it is safe because it's grown organic with no pesticides.

My grandchildren absolutely love my Kale Chips. It's a fun project we do together, from picking the kale in the garden, to preparation and enjoying it.

KALE CHIPS

Ingredients:

- Organic kale, 1 bunch
- 2 tbsp. olive oil
- Bragg's Liquid Aminos (comes in a spray bottle)
- Himalayan pink sea salt

Directions:

Tear kale in pieces, put in bowl, pour olive oil on kale, and stir. Place kale on cookie sheet, spread evenly, spray Bragg's Liquid Aminos on kale, and cover lightly. Sprinkle sea salt on to taste. Bake at 350 for 10 to 15 minutes. Take a peek after 10 minutes and adjust temperature accordingly—some ovens my run a little hot. Take out of oven when slightly crispy. If it's turning brown, turn down temperature.

This is a very quick easy snack for adults and children of all ages. Kale is known for being good for the eyes and macular degeneration. It is also packed with vegetable protein and minerals.

Bragg Liquid Aminos are amino acids—a liquid protein source

Himalayan sea salt is referred to as the purest salt in the world. Himalayan pink salt comes from the heart of the Himalayan Mountains. With hues of pink, red, and white, these vibrant colors are a sign of this salt's rich and varying mineral content.

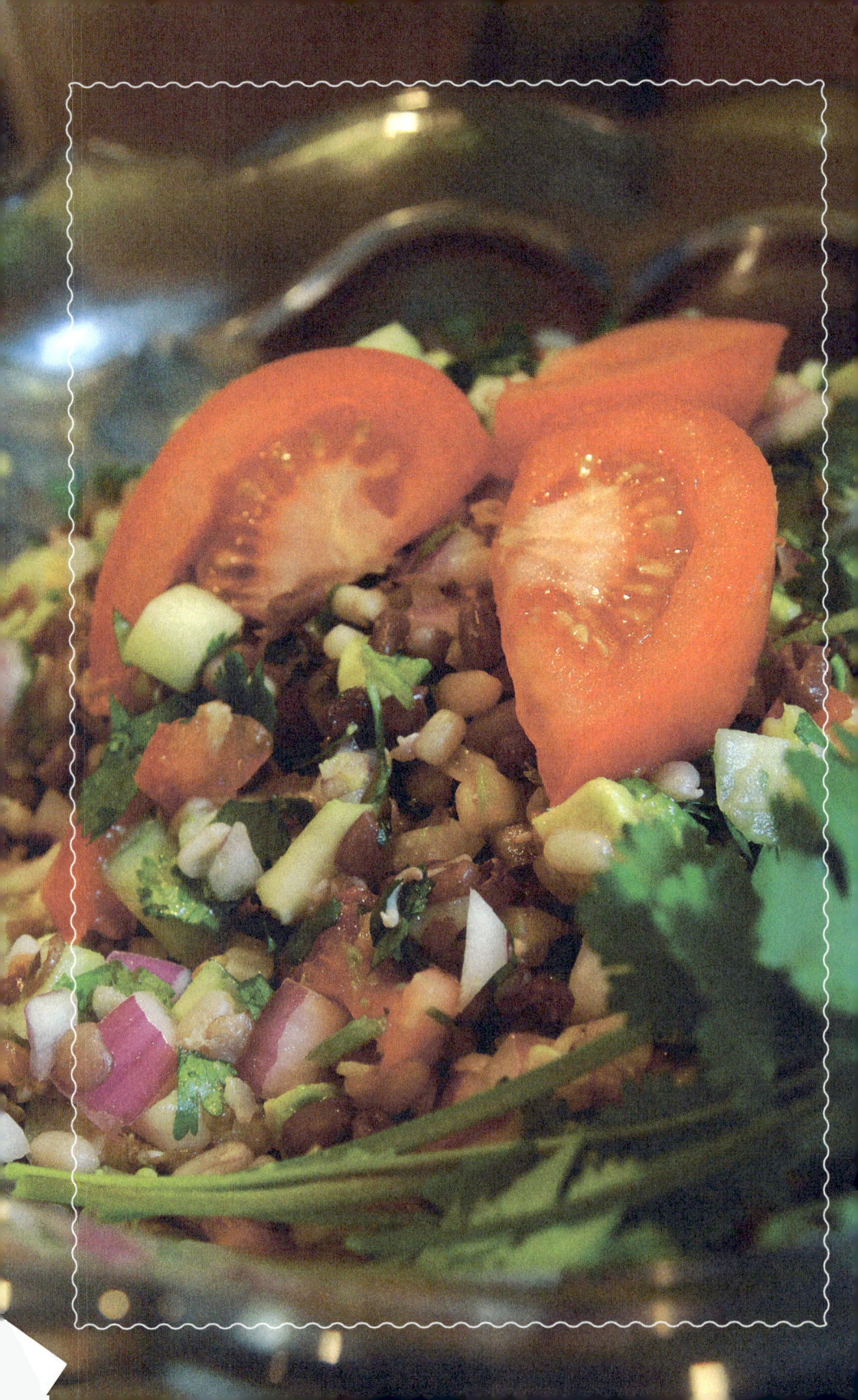

ORGANIC SPROUTED BEAN TRIO SUMMER SALAD

Serves 4

Ingredients:

- 1 organic red onion, chopped
- 1 organic cucumber, peeled and chopped
- 1 organic avocado, chopped
- 1 organic tomato, chopped, a few slices for the top for color
- 1 bunch of organic cilantro, chopped
- Himalayan pink sea salt to taste
- 1 organic lemon, squeezed
- 4 tbsp. of olive oil
- 1/8 tsp. of ground cumin (optional)
- 1 cup of true roots organic sprouted bean trio (Costco)

Directions:

Combine 1 cup of sprouted beans in 3 cups of water in a medium saucepan. Bring to boiling over medium heat. Reduce to low, cover, and simmer 5 minutes. Remove from heat and let stand, covered, for 10 minutes. Drain as needed.

Combine sprouted beans, red onion, cucumber, and cilantro and mix together. Pour on olive oil and lemon juice and salt to taste. Fold in tomatoes and avocado. Use some cilantro and tomato slices to garnish. Place in a nice serving bowl and enjoy.

This is light yet satisfying. I take this with me to parties—a healthy dish everyone loves. This salad is a great protein source. Every 1/3 cup serving of these beans contain 11 grams of protein.

COMPILED BY **HEATHER EDEN**

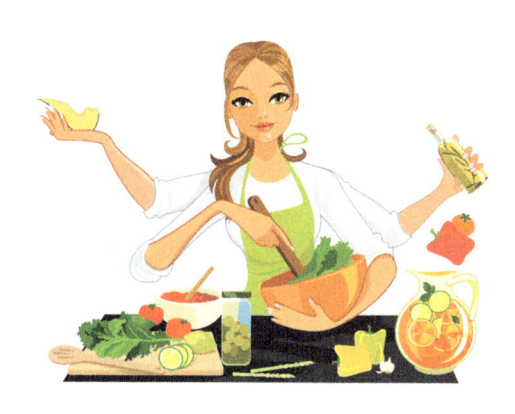

Kasie Roads, CHHP, AADP

I am an insatiable explorer, intuitive listener, and master illuminator—shining a brilliant light on my client's grand vision for their wellbeing and physical health. As a certified holistic health practitioner, I work with women who achieve results by tapping into their own innate wisdom. I believe you know yourself better than anyone, and honor your self-awareness by creating a custom plan to guide your exploration. I've spent the past twenty years on my own wellness journey, exploring a maze of healing modalities so I can now cherry-pick the juiciest, most delectable nuggets for you. All women deserve an opportunity to recharge through retreat and reflection. My passion is to chart the course and copilot your amazing adventure.

- www.wildrootwellness.com
- wildrootwellness@gmail.com

PRACTICE 25

Culturally Interconnected

By Kasie Roads, CHHP, AADP

Even into my late twenties, I was completely oblivious to the wonder of fermented foods. Sure, I'd seen plenty of pale, soggy sauerkraut adorning kielbasas, served to ruddy-faced men in lederhosen, but my diet was nearly kielbasa-free and I saw no other reason to be enticed.

At thirty, however, sauerkraut found me beyond the walls of the *biergarten* and we began our flirtation. Shopping at my favorite local health food store, I would see dozens of jars on the refrigerator shelves and be entranced by the variety and ridiculous price of shredded cabbage. "How can cabbage cost so much?" I would think. "It must be magical, or at least amazing!" So I read the ingredients. Cabbage, sea salt, arame, wakame, ginger, lactobacillus...hmmm? And I put it back on the shelf.

Then one day I saw it—a new brand of sauerkraut from the Cultured Pickle Shop in Berkeley. And it was HOT PINK—a rich and brilliant hot pink. I snatched the jar right up, took it home, and experienced love at first bite. As it turned out, fermented foods weren't just a side dish for sausage and schnitzel. In fact, its delightfully complex flavor arose from a harmonious synergy of tangy cabbage, earthy beets, crunchy carrot, and something undeniably larger than the sum of its parts. I was hooked.

Cultured foods are wondrous. In a nutshell, you take everyday ingredients, leave them out in non-refrigerated conditions, and allow bacteria to consume them. We then consume the bacteria and the leftover veggies they munched on. This process of fermenting creates a totally new food, birthed by the symbiotic relationship between the bacteria and the ingredients. The result? A highly digestible, and in most cases, probiotic-rich delicacy.

So, why should you consider incorporating aged cabbage as an esteemed condiment on your next plate?

Adding fermented foods to your diet:

- Strengthens your immune system.
- Re-inoculates your gut with healthy bacteria.
- Supports healing of conditions like irritable bowel syndrome or chronic diarrhea.
- Reduces cravings for sugar and processed foods.
- Inspires food adventure. The sheer variety of cultured delicacies will ensure an enlightened palate.
- Promotes your mission to eat healthy whole foods and increase nutrient density in your diet.
- Is as easy as you need it to be. Buy premade varieties or experiment with small batches in your kitchen.

There is yet another facet to this love I have for cultured foods—a philosophical and biological fascination for the bacteria themselves. Scientists now tell us that we're more bacteria than human and indicate that the gut appears to function as a second brain, bringing a new, scientifically-supported relevance to the phrase "Trust your gut." As taught by Joshua Rosenthal of the Institute for Integrative Nutrition, what we ingest builds our blood—the substance that creates and sustains our bodies. What a simple yet powerful concept, because all joking aside, who wants the quality of their body and mind built courtesy of Doritos and Diet Coke?

While the number of Microbiome studies have recently exploded, providing a metric ton of information to sift through, what's clear is the following:

The best strategy towards maintaining our health is to preserve and fortify our existing microbiological force field (i.e. the beneficial microbes on and in our skin). Think of bacteria, like lactobacillus, as your own personal micro Spartacus. If you're lucky, it's all over your skin and inside your body, fighting on your behalf to keep the bad stuff out! Provide a healthy terrain for the beneficial bacteria and they'll repay you by not allowing disease and illness to take residence in your body.

Support them by:

- Minimizing antibiotics and following their use with a period of probiotic re-inoculation.
- Discriminating with soap use. Many soaps and body care products wipe out the good bacteria on our skin. Your skin needs its natural oils to provide a good environment for healthy bacteria. Avoid ingredients like triclosan and alcohol.
- Following up a shower by rubbing high quality oils into your skin—like coconut, jojoba, or almond oil. Without a good filter in your showerhead, your skin is being dried out and damaged by chlorine, medications, and other chemicals in tap water.

As a philosophical concept, the word "culture" also provides ample intrigue. We know our attitudes, values, ideals, and beliefs are greatly influenced by our culture. When I think culture, I envision creative expressions of life experience through music, art, food, performance, and dance. These expressions allow us to feel human connection and inspiration. On the macro level, we see cultural characteristics within a family or society or even a global community. But as I was fascinated to learn from Daniel Vitalis, a leader in the Rewilding movement, the same thing is happening on a microscopic level! As we ingest food, water, and air, and interact through physical contact with people and the places we travel, so do we add their microbes to our own internal biological culture. It is a constant process spanning throughout our lives whereby we ingest and assimilate all we come into contact with. These interactions build who we are from the inside out. When we look at life from this perspective, it begs the question "What and whose bacteria do I want contributing to my physical and emotional health?"

I hope by sharing my own journey, I've inspired reflection on how culturally interconnected we truly are. As a human you have the opportunity to enhance the bacterial richness of our world by healthfully culturing yourself and sharing your culture with the rest of us.

SIMPLE SAUERKRAUT

The cornerstone of fermented foods. Here is a simple recipe to get you started:

Ingredients:

- 1 head green cabbage, sliced very thinly (reserve 2 large leaves)
- 2 to 3 carrots, grated
- 3 to 4 raw red beets, peeled and grated
- 2 tbs. sea salt (the good stuff)

Optional Embellishments:

- 1 tsp. caraway, mustard, or fennel seeds, lightly crushed
- Grated ginger, 1-inch piece (peeled)
- Grated green apple (peel skin)

Directions:

Process vegetables as outlined above and place into a large bowl. Sprinkle sea salt on top along with chosen embellishments. Wash hands.

Mix together all ingredients by hand, squeezing vegetables to break them down. The vegetables will feel much softer and begin to get juicy. Squeeze and mix for 5 minutes.

Pack the veggies into a 1-quart, wide-mouthed Mason jar. For each inch or two of kraut, take a moment to press the vegetables down, allowing the juice to rise above. Use a smaller Mason jar, wooden spoon, or kraut pounder to press the vegetables down, tightly packing them in. When you near the top, your liquid should be higher than the vegetables.

When the jar is full, use the reserved cabbage leaves to apply pressure on the kraut mixture and keep it submerged. If you have a lid with an airlock, use this, otherwise you can simply place a paper towel over the top and use a rubber band around the mouth of the jar to secure. It's important to let the kraut breathe while it ferments.

Leave at room temperature for about 5 to 10 days. Check daily to ensure the vegetables are staying submerged, pushing down if needed. If you see any foamy scum, simply skim it off.

Start tasting it on the third day. When it tastes good to you, put a regular lid on the Mason jar and store in the refrigerator. Sauerkraut will last many months in your refrigerator.

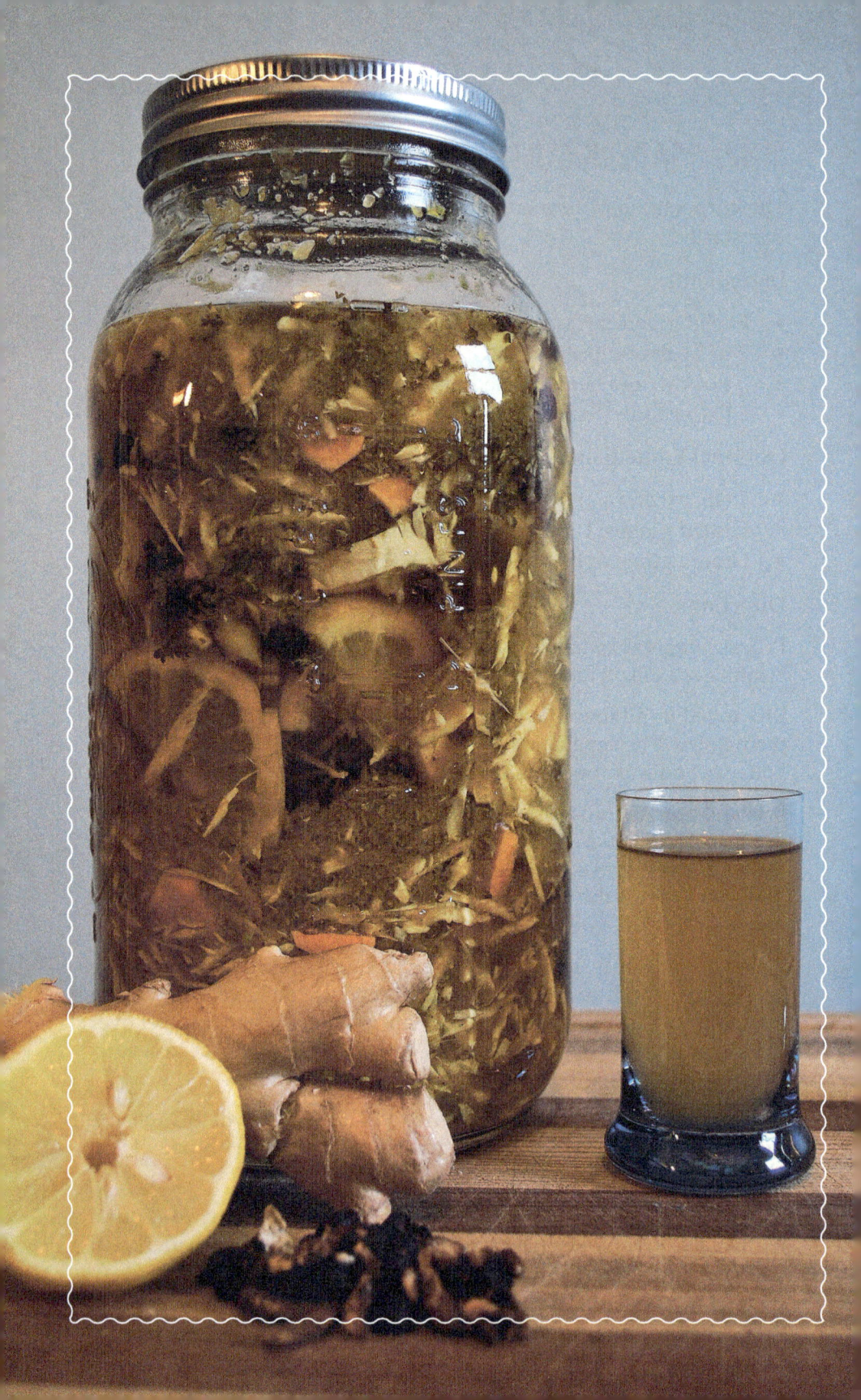

FIRE CIDER

The name alone is intriguing enough to inspire experimentation with this wonderfully versatile herbal remedy. Once you try this spicy, sweet, and pungent full-body warming elixir, you'll want a batch on hand for times when a cold, flu, or an overly celebratory night ails you. The ingredients are used for their digestive, stimulating, immune-boosting, anti-inflammatory, antibacterial, antiviral, decongestant, and circulatory boosting properties. Fire cider is also a unique secret ingredient for amazing fresh juices, salad dressings, stir-fry, marinades, soups, and steamed vegetables.

Ingredients:

- 2 onions, sliced
- 4 jalapenos, sliced
- 1/2 cup horseradish, grated
- 1 1/2 lemons, sliced with peels
- 2 fingers fresh ginger, sliced
- Cayenne to taste (try 1/8 to 1/4 tsp.)
- Honey to taste (start with 1/4 cup)
- Apple cider vinegar, enough to fill container

Optional embellishments: rosemary sprigs, turmeric (fresh if available), thyme, rosehips, ginseng, orange, grapefruit, schizandra berries, astragalus, parsley, burdock, oregano, peppercorns, cinnamon (Ceylon), and cardamom

Directions:

Chop garlic, onions, and jalapenos into small pieces. Grate fresh ginger and horseradish. Add desired embellishments.

Place into a wide-mouth quart jar and cover by 2 to 3 inches with apple cider vinegar. Add cayenne.

If using a metal lid, place a piece of parchment or wax paper between the jar and the lid to prevent corrosion from the vinegar. Shake well.

Let the jar sit in a cool, dark place for 3 to 6 weeks. Shake whenever you remember.

After one month, use cheesecloth to strain out the pulp, pouring the vinegar into a clean jar. Add honey.

For daily use, take 1 tablespoon. At first sign of cold, cough, or flu take 3 tablespoons.

Refrigerate and use within a year.

COMPILED BY **HEATHER EDEN**

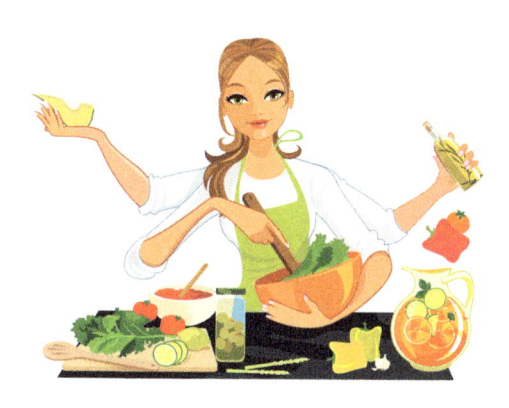

Suzi Pannenbacker, CHHC, AADP

Suzi Pannenbacker, also known as "wellness warriorette" has been a celebrity make-up artist and hair designer for over twenty years in Hollywood. She is also a certified holistic health and wellness coach (CHHC), and a member of AADP, Association of Drugless Practitioners.

Suzi has also been certified professionally as a raw chef and instructor, and has extensive training in aromatherapy and healing with essential oils, incorporating them in food, beauty products, and wellbeing.

Also, becoming an international advisory consultant for Japanese Superfoods Association, she has become a complete facilitator for transforming people's health, wellness, and beauty on the inside and out.

- www.wellnesswarriorette.com
- suzi@wellnesswarriorette.com
- www.facebook.com/wellnesswarriorette
- www.facebook.com/suzipannenbacker

PRACTICE 26

Freedom Within

By Suzi Pannenbacker, CHHC, AADP

I would like to shed some light on a pure "freedom within" for all of you out there maybe battling with this issue. I battled having freedom my whole life, searching and trying the newest, latest, and supposed greatest diet of the month! It confused me greatly, but I continued with conviction to find the "perfect" one.

There was always a new way of eating to be healthy, or getting rid of this bulge, or getting radiant skin and making your eyes sparkle, or getting more energy, or how about making him love you more! Any of these sound familiar?

We, as women (especially if desperate) will try anything, and may I add, will spend any amount—even it if means taking out a second mortgage—to make ourselves radiant, sparkly, and more desirable…right?

In my late teen years, the neurosis began. I bought teen magazines and fashion magazines that taught us about having an image physically impossible for most. On top of that, there were multiple diets, workout regiments, beauty tips, hairstyles and makeup tips, and "make the boys go crazy" tips! How hard could all this be? "Piece of cake!" I thought—which by the way, you can't have—and the path of destruction began, without me ever knowing it!

By the time I was twenty-five, I was a lifetime member at four gyms. I was already thin, but I didn't look like what the magazines showed me. So I thought I could go to the gym and mold my body into the perfect image, as they promised I would be able to do.

I also wanted to be tan, have perfect skin, long hair, different colored eyes, and the list goes on. I was a prisoner in my own body, and mostly my mind, and didn't even know it!

I was everything short of perfect, and I was determined to figure out a way to be what the media made me believe I should be. This nonsense did not stop. In fact, it only got worse with age and with my chosen profession.

I became a cosmetologist and specialized in hair and makeup. I loved transforming people and helping them feel beautiful and special. I loved working with other people who had an image neurosis, too! We mirror the ones we are.

It all seemed so right, and no, I still was striving for my own satisfaction and perfection. But I was in an environment that was ever-changing and never satisfied, and I was always trying the latest and greatest new thing.

Then I landed an opportunity in Los Angeles and became a Celebrity Make-Up Artist to the rich and famous! I had arrived to the world of perfection—so I believed. This is where my real neurosis spun out of control. Anything was possible there, but it usually had a pretty hefty price tag attached to it. All the best of everything is in Hollywood. If you could dream it, it probably existed.

I worked a lot and always strove for more. I learned how to push myself to places that became dangerous. I suddenly wanted to be thinner, and have more energy, and always "be, look, and feel" more! Working long hours, and for many days, there was little time to go to the gyms (BTW: I had a lifetime membership). The only way to stay slim was to not eat, and energy came with lots of caffeine, or some other concoction or fad tonic.

It worked for a while. I got thinner than I had ever been. But basically I developed an eating disorder, along with over-exhaustion, blowing out my adrenals and having panic attacks on a daily basis. I was in a downward spiral. However, after being in Hollywood and learning how illusion worked, I mastered my own illusion and nobody knew I was a prisoner in my body and mind. I learned not to walk and live in my truth. I was surviving, but not living, and I had no peace.

I prayed for help from God and asked for guidance and direction. Let me tell you, when He answers prayers, it may not be the way you think it will be answered. I resisted and fought with the direction He was leading me, but ultimately I knew it was right.

It started with my diet. I started eating healthier, plant-based and raw foods. I stopped all caffeine of any kind, and I stopped eating processed foods. I loved how I was feeling, and this passion led me to become a certified holistic health coach. I also became a certified raw plant-based chef. I am now certified to make my celebrity clients not only beautiful on the outside but gorgeous on the inside!

Through my education and transformation, I have learned that there is no "perfect." How liberating to stop chasing something that does not exist. I have also learned something called bio-individuality, which means: what is good for one person, may not serve another the same way. Our bodies are unique.

I have found my Inner Freedom, and I now share with others how to achieve theirs. Finding what serves you well and makes you feel good, healthy, and balanced creates a fulfilled life and a happy way to live. When you love yourself enough to accomplish this task and discover your light, you become a path for others to follow and become the leader you were born to be.

I am including two of my favorite "go-to" recipes. Both are raw, nutritiously delicious, and simple to make. No fancy equipment needed—and kid-friendly! I call the entree dish "Cup of Thai." The other recipe is called "Mojo Mites." I hope you enjoy.

Peace and Freedom Be With You....

These bites I call Mojo Mites are packed full of nutrition but taste like a dessert! They are loaded with chocolate and superfoods to give a burst of natural energy and chewiness that is sure to please everyone!

A great breakfast to go, or pick-me-up mid-afternoon, or a treat for kids!

MOJO MITES

Yield: 50 balls, depending on size

Ingredients:

- 1/2 cup raw cashews
- 1/2 cup raw almonds (optional to soak and dehydrate, but not required)
- 3 cups of pitted soft dates
- 1/2 cup raw cacao powder
- 2 tbsp. chia seeds
- 3/4 cup raw shelled hemp seeds
- 6 tbsp. raw sweetened cacao nibs
- 1 tbsp. Maca powder
- 2 tsp. mesquite powder
- 2 tbsp. raw sprouted pumpkin seeds
- 1 tsp. vanilla
- 1/8 tsp. Himalayan salt
- * 1 to 4 drops Young Living Essential Oils, — peppermint or orange
- 3 to 4 tbsp. finely chopped macadamia nuts
- 1/3 cup raw dried Goji berries, coarsely chopped (or dried fruit of choice)

Directions:

Put all ingredients except chopped nuts and dried fruit in large food processor with S blade and process until a coarse and pliable dough forms. If it seems dry, (usually from dates lack of moisture), add a bit of water a few drops at a time until it all pulls together.

Now add the chopped nuts and fruit and pulse to combine.

Roll into balls and place on sheet. Refrigerate, and when firm, place in container. Can also be put in the freezer.

You can easily cut recipe in half — but you will want these babies around for easy access!

*Note: Only use Young Living Essential Oils for Internal Consumption. 100 percent Therapeutic Grade

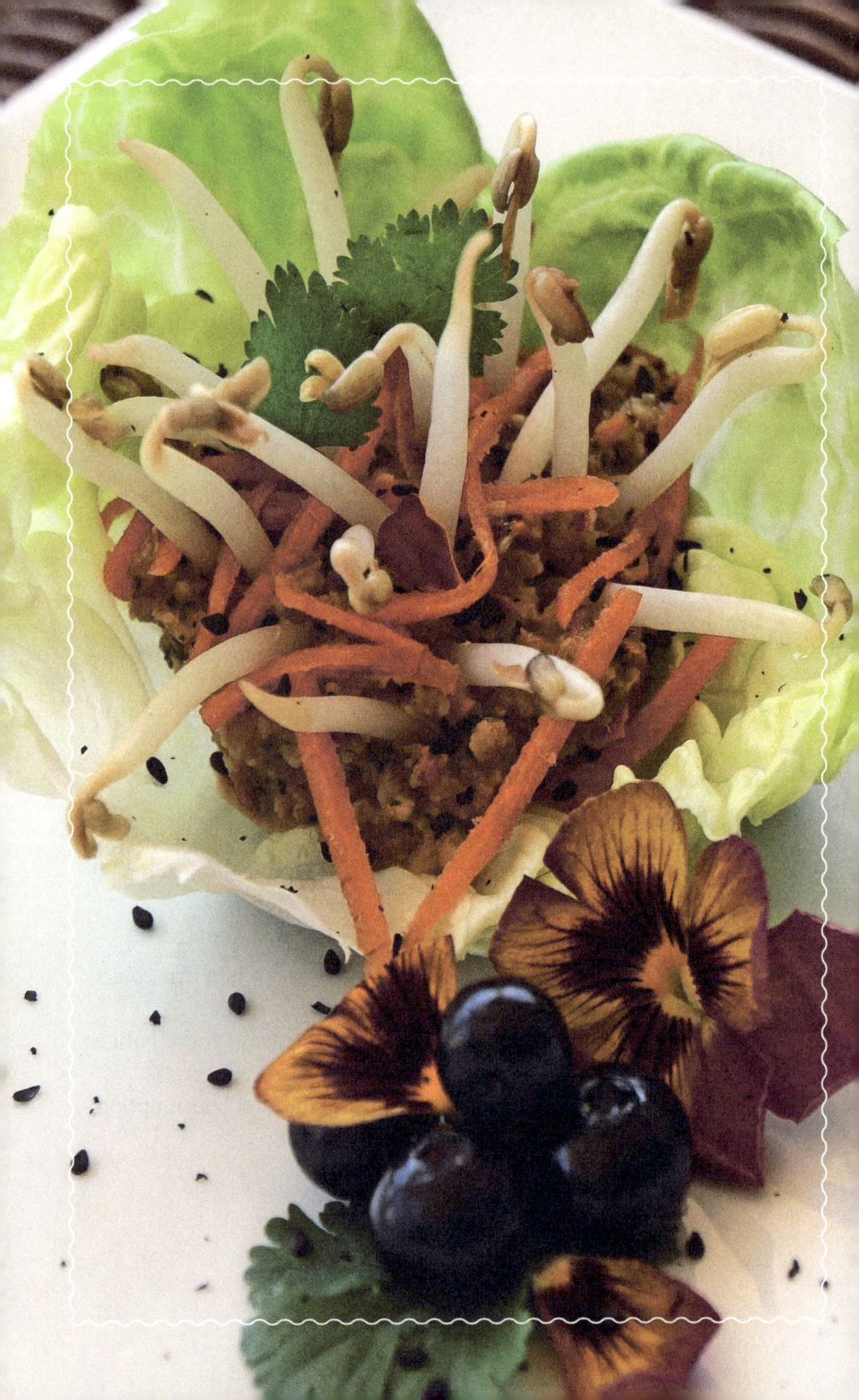

COMPILED BY **HEATHER EDEN**

CUP OF THAI

I call this recipe "Cup of Thai!" It is a raw version of Asian-inspired lettuce cups. Sweet, spicy, and delicious! It's fun for the family to make at the table and build to order for each serving. Hope you enjoy these as much as my friends and I do!

Serves 4

Prepare ingredients and set aside:

- 1 1/2 cups raw walnuts (optional to soak and dehydrate, but not required)
- 1/2 cup carrots, diced
- 1/2 cup red bell pepper, diced
- 1/2 cup celery, diced
- 1/4 cup green scallions, minced
- 1/2 cup fresh cilantro, minced

Garnish:

- 1 head of butter lettuce
- 3/4 cups fresh mung beans, sprouted
- 3/4 cups carrots, grated
- Cilantro leaves
- Directions:
- Pull apart, wash, and dry lettuce leaves to make cups.
- Place on tray.
- Place mung beans and grated carrots in separate dishes for easy access.

Sauce:

- 1/4 cup namu shoyu - gluten free
- 1/4 cup raw honey
- 1 tsp. grated fresh ginger
- 1 tbsp. hulled sesame seeds
- 1 tsp. fresh garlic, minced
- 1 tsp. red pepper flakes
- 1 tbsp. sesame oil (note: I like toasted sesame oil better, but it is not raw. My Freedom Within lets me be OK with this!)

Directions:

In a food processor with an S blade, combine all sauce ingredients until incorporated.

Add walnuts and pulse 4 to 5 times until it looks like a meat texture.

Add rest of prepared ingredients and pulse lightly 4 to 5 times, still keeping chunky. Do not over process!

Place in bowl and serve with garnishes.

Place a lettuce leaf on plate and put a spoonful of "meat" in cup. Top with mung beans, grated carrots, and cilantro.

COMPILED BY **HEATHER EDEN**

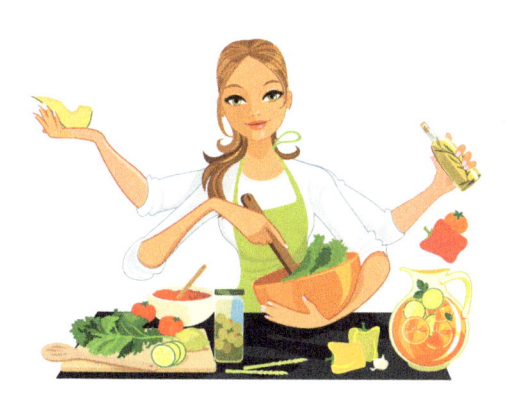

Kasia Cummings, CHHC, AADP

Kasia Cummings, CHHC, AADP, is a certified holistic health coach and beauty entrepreneur, holding degrees in medicinal chemistry and holistic nutrition. Her two companies, Whole Health Evolution and Buffalo Gal Organics, are the perfect pairing of science and nature, woven with spirit, alchemy, and love. Through Whole Health Evolution, she works with people in all walks of life to manifest their true path—to love their bodies with soul-centered counsel, in a natural, holistic, and spiritual way. Her holistic and organic skincare company, Buffalo Gal Organics, is an eco-conscious bath, body, and beauty line that is vegan, organic, and infused with healing energy.

Reach out to Kasia Here:

- www.facebook.com/BuffaloGalOrganics
- www.facebook.com/WholeHealthEvolution
- www.twitter.com/BfloGalOrganics
- www.BuffaloGalOrganics.com
- www.BuffaloGalOrganics.etsy.com
- www.holeHealthEvolution.com/blog

PRACTICE 27

Unraveling the Fat Myth

By Kasia Cumming, CHHC, AADP

How many times have you heard this? Fat makes you fat. I've lived this fallacy for a good portion of my life, eating fat-free this and low-fat that because I thought I was doing my body a favor. Fat was the enemy and I was determined to be fat-free forever. Butter on those veggies? No! Olive oil on your salad? I think not! I was determined to stave off all those pounds, but unfortunately for me, I was doing just the opposite…I was gaining weight even though I was eating "healthy." Thankfully, as I was getting my undergrad degree in medicinal chemistry, a great little course in biochemistry changed the way I looked at what I was putting into my body. Fat was no longer a four letter word!

So let's talk a little about the basics of why fat IS good for you. Fats are an essential part of cell function, helping to repair cell walls and keeping membranes pliable. They transport vitamins through the body and assist in their metabolism, as well as helping to keep the body warm and creating ready energy for times of great stress. It's interesting that we've vilified fat when it's an essential component that is necessary for our survival. Our DNA calls for it, our brains need it to develop, and our organs use it to protect their basic functions.

As we look at the types of fat that we can consume, we do need to address good fats versus bad fats. One of the reasons that fat has gotten such a bad reputation is due to the overconsumption of processed, prepackaged, deep fried foods laden with saturated and trans fats. Biologically, these bad fats break down in our bodies and form free radicals and disrupt DNA function, causing cell death. Something to think about the next time you eat that deep fried processed thing you found in a box! Read your labels and choose foods that contain Monounsaturated Fatty Acids (MUFA) or Polyunsaturated Fatty Acids (PUFA). These are the healthy fats that help your body perform at its optimum efficiency.

Ok, so why are these MUFAs and PUFAs so good for us? These fats have been a staple of the human diet for thousands of years. Think back to the popularity of the Mediterranean Diet and why so many loved it. It was because their bodies felt satiated due to the inclusion of healthy fats...everyday! Staples of the diet included olives and olive oil, nuts, seeds, fatty fish such as salmon—all of which added not only healthy fat but also trace minerals, vitamins, and antioxidants. Their bodies responded because they were eating nutrient-dense foods. The by-product? They lost weight, had more energy, and radiated a healthy glow.

Now, after all this talk about adding in healthy, you might be wondering how you can add these tasty bits of love into your diet. Here are a few examples to get you started:

1. Fatty fish: salmon, tuna, trout, mackerel. These fish are traditionally found in cold water and contain high levels of Omega 3, 6, and 9, which are essential for maintaining proper weight and lowering cholesterol.

2. Olives/olive oil: a great source of healthy triglycerides and Omega 9, which helps to protect the heart. EVOO also has high levels of polyphenols that act as antioxidants in the bloodstream.

3. Flax seeds: very high in Omega 3 and also a great source of fiber. If you are vegan, you can use this as an egg substitute when cooking. One thing to remember: flax must be freshly ground to retain its benefits and absorptive properties. Eating it whole will do nothing for you! Flax can also go rancid, so refrigerate, especially if you buy flax oil.

4. Almonds/nuts/seeds: Most nuts and seeds are high in trace minerals, such as selenium, copper, and magnesium, in addition to the high level of good fats. A handful is a perfect portion.

5. Avocados: Although they are calorie-dense, avocadoes are a perfect way to get your fats! Use them in dressings that call for dairy to make them vegan, add to a wrap for a great vegetarian option, or even broil them with eggs—delicious!

6. Coconut oil: Here is the one exception to the rule on saturated fats. Coconut oil is high in essential fatty acids and sincerely is one of the best detoxifiers in this world. You can eat it straight up as a butter substitute, use it for oil pulling for oral health, as a cooking oil, and topically as a natural moisturizer. And studies have shown that the consumption of EVCO (extra virgin coconut oil) lessens and reverses the symptoms of Alzheimer's.

The above list is not inclusive, of course, but it will get you on the right track to adding in healthy fats to your diet. It's easier than you think and a simple swap for olive or coconut oil versus processed, hydrogenated oils could be the perfect start in the right direction!

As we wrap up, I'll leave you with a few things…

Always read labels! Become familiar with what's really in your food and know the difference between an ingredient statement and ingredient deck.

Small changes make for lasting results. Each week, try something new and use up what you have in your pantry then replace it with a healthier option. You'll be less wasteful, healthier, and save some money, too!

The perfect ratio of Omega 3 to Omega 6 is 2:1. If you are looking to add Omegas in as a supplement then make sure it has this ratio. Strive for 1000mg per day. Read the label and buy the best you can afford.

Buy organic whenever you can! The less toxic load your body has to process the better it will assimilate nutrients. Give your body its best fighting chance!

Sending you love and blessings!

Namaste,

Kasia

THE BEST EVER PUMPKIN MUFFINS

These tasty treats are vegan, gluten-free, and dairy-free!

Ingredients:

- 1 can organic pumpkin
- 1/2 cup coconut oil
- 1/2 cup organic applesauce
- 1/4 cup flaked coconut
- 1/4 cup chia seeds
- 1/2 cup chopped walnuts (or any other nut)
- 1/2 cup dried cranberries
- 3/4 cup vegan chocolate chips
- 1 1/4 cup coconut flour
- 1 1/4 cup almond meal flour
- 1/2 cup quinoa flakes
- 1 tsp. baking soda
- 1 tsp. baking powder
- 1 tbsp. cinnamon
- 1/2 cup raw honey or maple syrup
- 1 tsp. vanilla

Directions:

Preheat oven to 350 degrees.

Combine all dry ingredients (coconut flour, almond flour, baking soda, baking powder, cinnamon, chia seeds) together and mix thoroughly or sift together with a sifter and set aside.

Mix together canned pumpkin, honey or maple syrup (for the vegan version), vanilla, and applesauce. Melt the coconut oil gently so that it is liquid and add to the mix. Stir thoroughly.

Combine wet and dry mixes then fold in all other ingredients, including chocolate chips, cranberries, and nuts. Your mixture should be thick and not super wet. If you find that it is really dry looking, you can add some additional applesauce (up to 1/2 cup) or one ripe mashed banana and stir together.

Fill lined muffin tins 3/4 full and bake for 25 to 30 minutes or until toothpick comes out clean. Let cool and serve.

You can add or omit ingredients, such as nuts, if allergic. My kids love these muffins (while not loving pumpkin or coconut), so even your pickiest eater may just fall in love with these!

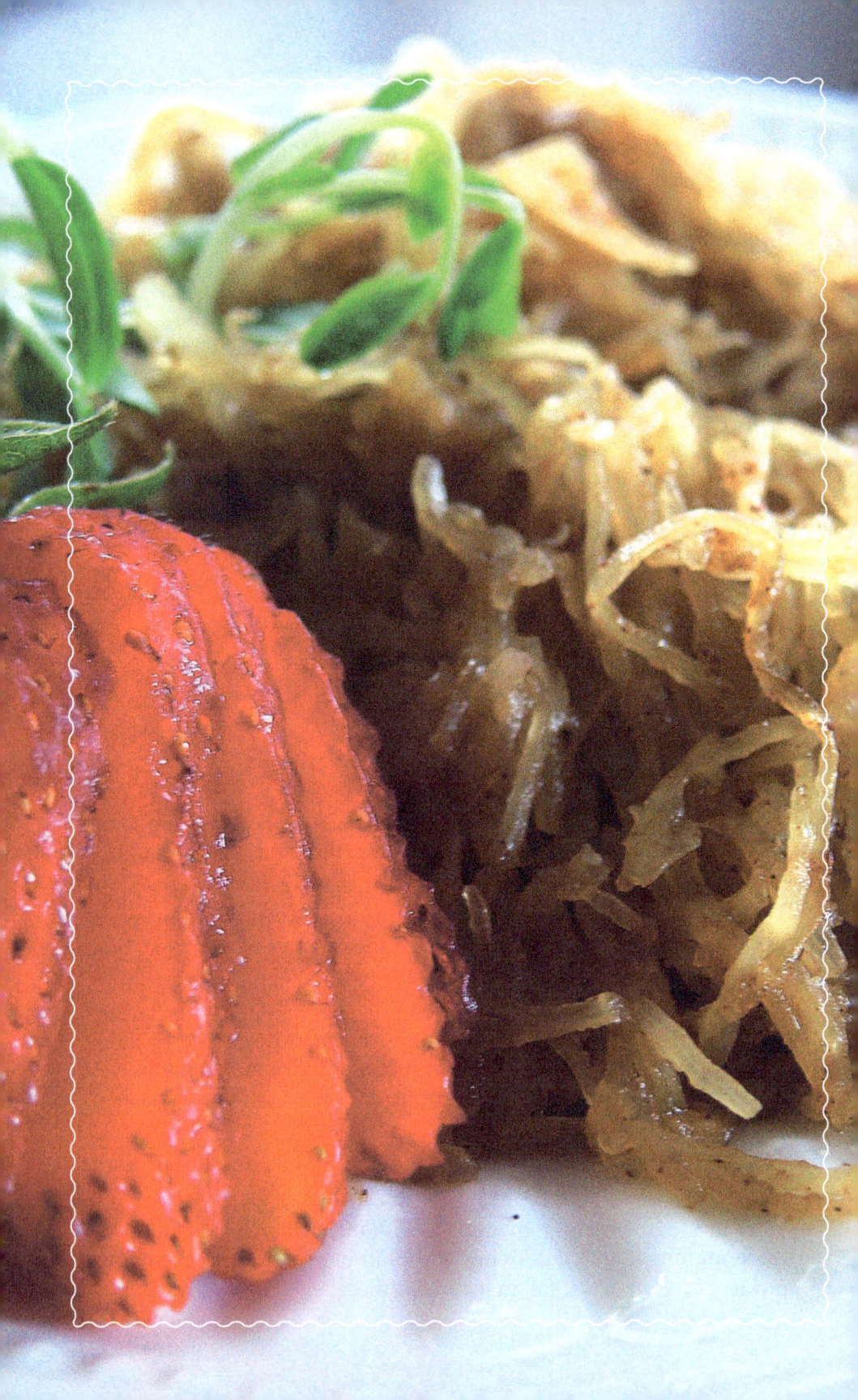

SWEET FRIED SPAGHETTI SQUASH

Whether you eat this as a tasty (and healthy) dessert or as something new for breakfast, this spaghetti squash recipe is a perfect alternative to traditional carb-laden pasta.

This recipe is vegan, gluten-free, and dairy-free.

Ingredients:

- 1 small spaghetti squash
- 1/4 cup maple syrup (or raw honey for non-vegans)
- 2 tsp. ground cinnamon
- 1 to 2 tbsp. Coconut oil
- 1/4 cup chopped walnuts
- Fresh fruit to garnish, such as blueberries or strawberries

To prepare squash:

Cut spaghetti squash in half and scoop out seeds with a spoon. Place face down on a glass dish and bake at 350 degrees for about 20 to 30 minutes, until tender. Remove from the oven and let cool then take a fork to scoop out squash flesh to form spaghetti strands. In a hurry? You can microwave the squash halves in a glass dish for 6 to 8 minutes for each half.

Directions:

Melt coconut oil in pan (if you have a small squash, you can use a bit less oil than the 2 tbsp. mentioned above to keep a healthy fat ratio).

Add in shredded squash and heat up. Allow the pieces to get crispy and stir frequently to prevent burning.

Add in maple syrup and cinnamon just before you are ready to serve, stirring thoroughly. Top with chopped walnuts (optional) and enjoy!

COMPILED BY **HEATHER EDEN**

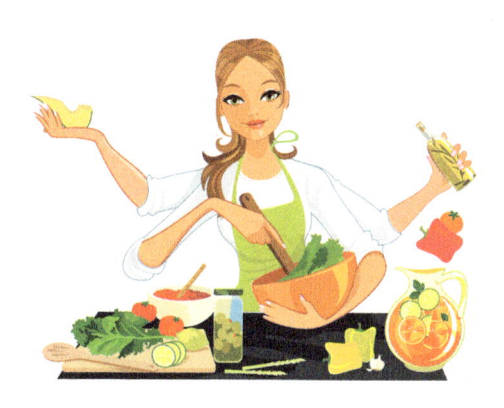

Stephanie Locricchio, CHHC, AADP

Stephanie Locricchio is a graduate of the Institute for Integrative Nutrition and is certified by the American Association of Drugless Practitioners.

As a multitasking "Mompreneur," she wears many hats: licensed esthetician, speaker, writer, and food activist. Her mission is to raise awareness on issues that impact health and wellness. Through education, she empowers people to make better choices on food and personal care products. She offers a clean living program that has assisted hundreds in reaching their health goals and recovering from food related disorders.

Through her work, Stephanie has built a team of wellness warriors on a mission to impact change and create a cleaner, healthier future, proving that there is power in numbers. Together, they are assisting others to step into their power to live a prosperous, clean, and balanced lives.

- ✉ slocricchio@gmail.com
- 🏠 www.stephanielocricchio.com
- 🏠 www.wellnesswarriorsunite.com
- f www.facebook.com/stephanie.locricchio
- f www.facebook.com/wellnesswarriorsunite

PRACTICE 28

A Legacy of Health

By Stephanie Locricchio, CHHC, AADP

Eating is a culture, and our relationship with food is formed during childhood. Habits are made to be broken and my story is proof that education can change everything. My nickname growing up was the "Häagen Dazs queen." I loved sweets, treats, and soda. As children, we don't fully understand that every action has a direct effect on our health, mood, and energy. Growing up, I was a product of the Standard American Diet. My shift began as a young adult when I attended esthetics school. I learned about the toxic ingredients in our personal care products and it prompted me to reevaluate my choices. I became savvy with reading ingredient labels and this practice carried over into all aspects of my life. I started to investigate the foods that entered my body. The discoveries about the food in this country disturbed me. My favorite pastime became reading health and wellness books. Knowledge is power and when you know better, you can do better. This quest for information had lasting and permanent effects on my relationship with food. The power of this knowledge led to a career change that has allowed me to touch the lives of my family, friends, community, and clients.

If the saying "You are what you eat" is true, what have we become? Most people would not describe themselves as fast, cheap, or fake, yet an alarming 62 percent of the calories we consume come from processed foods, while only 5 percent come from fruits and vegetables. Our supermarket shelves are lined with "food-like" substances laden with chemicals, GMOS, preservatives, and pesticides, making it almost impossible to locate actual food in the dozens of aisles. We live in a society of extreme couponing, and food shopping has become a bargain hunt. We are programmed by commercial advertisements to look for cost and convenience over quality and nutrition content. In the hustle and bustle of life, we are bombarded with convenience foods at every given turn—in gas stations and shopping malls. As a result, we live in a country that is sick, overweight, and looking for a miracle pill or diet to cure all our problems.

Calorie counting is a widely used practice for weight management, but what most people fail to realize is that calories are just one part of a bigger picture. The truth about the foods you consume are listed on the ingredient labels. Food companies use buzz marketing terms like "natural" and a "good source of whole grains" to draw you in. If you scratch just beneath the surface, you will be shocked to find artificial sweeteners, trans fats, and tons of sugar in the products we feed our children daily.

Today, mothers are faced with the unique challenge of raising the first generation of children that have a shorter life expectancy than their parents. The obesity epidemic in this country is trickling down to school-aged children and lifestyle choices are to blame. We're a busy society, working long hours, so convenience foods have become the standard for meals. It is rare that families sit down at the table to eat a home-cooked meal. Most families eat on the run, frequenting pizza shops, fast food restaurants, or cooking their meals in the microwave. The correlation between the rise of preventative illness in our children and the culture of eating in this country can't be denied. Mothers lead by example and set the tone for the family's relationship with food. Children mirror our behavior and often our words go unheard. We teach our children the fundamentals of life. Therefore, it's our responsibility to instill healthy habits in our growing children.

Developing a healthy relationship with food is a process that requires discipline and knowledge. It is important to be present and mindful at mealtime. When eating becomes an out-of-body experience, followed by feelings of guilt and shame, it's clearly time to make a change. Mindful eating and self-care create long-term lifestyle changes. Let's face it, diets don't work. It is a behavioral change for a temporary period of time to reach a specific goal. Once the diet ends, most people will go back to their old ways because no mindset shift has occurred on food choices. I have coached hundreds of clients to release unwanted pounds and find a healthy relationship with food. There are three key questions I recommend asking prior to a meal or a snack:

What am I eating? Where did it come from? What is it doing for my body?

When food is viewed as the vital fuel your body requires to thrive, suddenly the plate of fast food goes from delicious to toxic. The golden rule of health is to practice the 80/20 rule. Eighty percent of the food consumed should be providing nutrition and energy to our bodies. There is a wide variety of whole foods that can be enjoyed guilt-free, no calorie counting necessary. Twenty percent of the time, feel free to dine out, have a cocktail, or indulge in a sweet treat. This shift takes the guilt out of eating and the roller coaster of failed diets will finally be put to rest.

To achieve ultimate health, we must address the onslaught of toxins we are at battle with daily. Our body has become ground zero for toxins. Our food is nutritionally bankrupt due to the overwhelming amount of "'cides" (Latin term for death) used on the topsoil. Therefore, it's vital to fill in the gaps with supplementation and to have a system to cleanse the body of toxins. Mindful eating and nutritional cleansing are the cornerstones of my nutrition plan. Toxins create visceral fat, deplete our energy levels, and inhibit us from reaching our health goals. Your body is designed to feel good and heal itself. Once you cross over and feel the shift, you will never go back.

As moms, we tend to put ourselves last when we should be on the top of the priority list. Remember, a healthy mom creates a healthy family. Mothers are the heart of the family and our legacy lives on long after we are gone. Cooking creates a culture rich in tradition and recipes are passed on for generations. Mealtime is a special time to create memories and reflect on the day. Cherish this time and cook colorful meals to nourish your family.

Here are some tips to take the stress out of the kitchen:

Always meal plan for the week and cook in bulk so there are leftovers.

Create a peaceful and organized environment in your kitchen.

Involve your children in the kitchen; this is the best way to address picky eaters.

Cook using fresh ingredients and lots of love. Plant seeds of health and watch them grow!

Here are some simple recipes from my kitchen to yours:

HERB-STUFFED ARTICHOKES

Ingredients:

- 4 artichokes
- Favorite seasoning
- 1 1/2 tsp. garlic powder
- 1 tsp. salt
- 1 tsp. pepper
- 2 lemons
- 2 tbsp. fresh chopped parsley
- 2 tbsp. fresh chopped basil
- 2 tbsp. fresh chopped sage
- 16 cloves of garlic
- 1 tbsp. EVOO
- 3 cups of panko or gluten-free breadcrumbs

Directions:

Open the artichokes by turning them upside down and gently pressing down. Open leaves with your hands to allow room for the stuffing. Squeeze 1 1/2 lemon on the artichokes and rub the leaves with the lemon juice.

In a large bowl, mix the breadcrumbs, seasoning, salt, pepper, garlic powder, parsley, basil, sage, 12 cloves of garlic, olive oil and breadcrumb together.

In a large sauté pan, fill the pan with water middle of the way so half the artichoke is submerged in water. Squeeze the remaining lemon into the water and cut up the lemons you used and scatter them about in the pan. Crush the remaining 4 cloves of garlic and put them in the pan also.

Add the artichokes and cook covered over a medium flame for approximately 45 minutes. Allow to cool and serve immediately.

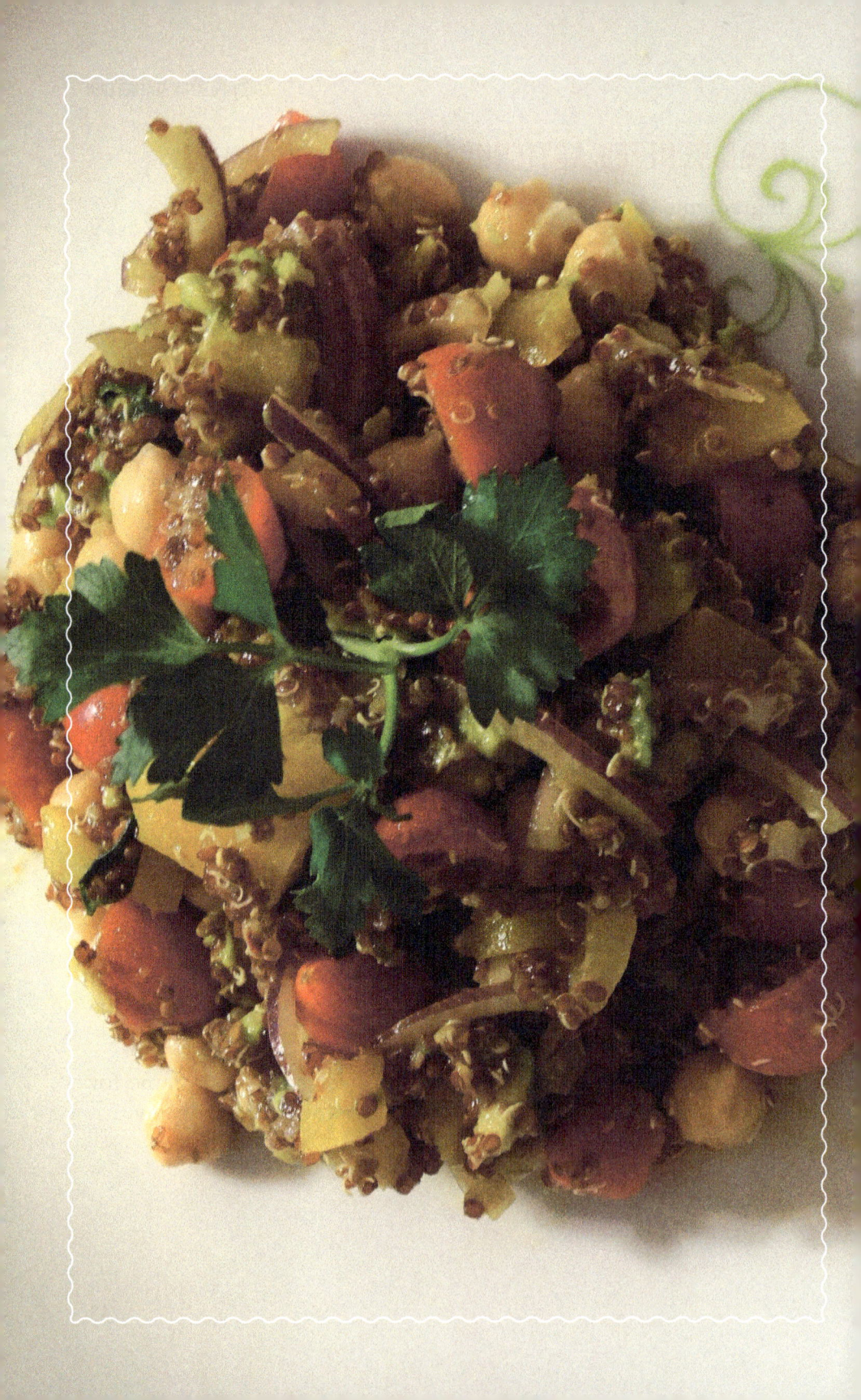

"EVERYTHING BUT THE KITCHEN SINK" QUINOA SALAD

Ingredients:

- 1 cup quinoa (rinsed)
- 2 cups of low-sodium vegetable broth
- 1 kombu sea vegetable (optional)
- 1 tbsp. EVOO
- 1 1/2 lemon
- Your favorite seasoning (Trader Joe's everyday seasoning)
- 1 1/2 tbsp. fresh parsley
- 1 1/2 cup organic cherry tomatoes, halved
- 1 small red onion, chopped
- 1 avocado, diced
- 1 yellow pepper, diced
- 1 cup chickpeas, rinsed
- 1 cup organic corn (optional)

Directions:

Rinse quinoa and combine with the vegetable broth and kombu in a saucepan. Bring to a boil, then cover and reduce to a low flame until water is absorbed about 15 minutes.

In the meanwhile, chop and prepare your vegetables.

When the quinoa has cooked thoroughly allow it to cool and fluff it with a fork. Remove and discard the Kombu.

Drizzle the olive oil and squeeze lemon on the cooked quinoa. Add your favorite seasoning to taste.

Combine all the vegetables and fresh herbs in a large bowl. Toss to mix and serve.

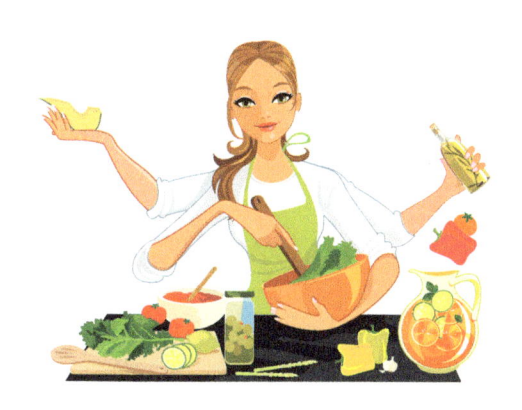

Jennifer Bain Smith, HLC, HC

Jennifer Bain Smith is a certified holistic lifestyle coach and a health coach. She received her training from the C.H.E.K. Institute and the Institute of Integrative Nutrition. She is also the founder of Fresh Start Nutrition and Coaching, LLC.

Based out of New York, Jennifer helps her clients learn to create a healthy relationship with food that allows them to eat in a way that supports their unique biochemistry and metabolism.

Jennifer's mission is to empower each of her clients to live the healthiest and happiest life possible using whole foods as the most important tool in the toolbox!

www.freshstartnutritionandcoaching.com

www.facebook.com/freshstartnutritionandcoaching

PRACTICE 29

We Are All In This Together

By Jennifer Bain Smith, HLC, HC

Walking around in your daily life as a mother, do you ever feel plain old out of control? I did for years, until I started to figure out that what we are eating and what our children are eating is actually what has become completely out of control!!

This thought process and some very real things that were happening within my immediate family started me on a journey towards a whole foods approach to mindful eating. How many of us spend hours shopping for the right healthy ingredients (or what we have been told are healthy) for our recipes and the best snacks to have on hand for our little ones and their precious friends? We ALL do, and yet we find ourselves frustrated again and again when our babies have asthma and cases of allergies tenfold of what we saw when we were children, not to mention any other number of ailments.

A simple experiment a couple of years ago led me to the most amazing discovery, the discovery that food really is our medicine. What we put into our bodies is incredibly important and where that food comes from packs just as much, if not more of a punch.

At one point in my life, I had a stye in my right eye for over a month. I had taken two rounds of antibiotics and was using an antibiotic cream, but nothing was working. The stye wouldn't go away. After the first month came and went, the stye had turned into what I would call a cyst and it was right in the center of my eyelid on the lash line (it was very difficult to use mascara and believe me…I cared about THAT!). Three months later, after hoping it would get better on its own, I decided to go back to the doctor. He told me that the only thing

I could do was to have it removed surgically. After leaving the office and going home to think about what he said, I decided to do nothing for a few more days but consider the situation. I really didn't want to have surgery on my eyelid.

During this same time, I had been looking for hidden sugars in my food and began eliminating processed food from my diet. I was beginning to feel so good day to day that I decided to eliminate everything I had been eating except organic fruit, organic vegetables, grass-fed/finished organic meats, and healthy fats. I made a commitment to myself to be very strict for thirty days and see how I would feel. So at this point, I was not having any grains or dairy—no caffeine either. The only thing I was drinking was water. This may seem over the top to some of you but at the time, I figured it was only thirty days, so why not give it a try?

Well, I had not been thinking of my stye in relation to the food I was eating so I was astounded when I woke up on the sixth day and it was completely gone! What had turned into a hard lump that was going to have to be surgically removed had completely disappeared on its own without medicine or surgery, four months after it had first appeared.

And so it began...a world full of whole foods and whole foods only. Although it may sound limiting at first, I felt as if a door had flown open and everything was brand new. I loved cooking and baking and my children were always in the kitchen with me. Now we were on an adventure. I started modifying almost every recipe I had and began creating new ones. I taught myself how to bake without sugar and flour, and guess what? It was fun!

I was enjoying myself so much that I started coaching other moms on how to move away from the Standard American Diet (SAD) or even the traditional food pyramid that we have so ingrained in us. My new clients were not only experiencing the same health benefits, stable mood, and great night's sleep that I was getting but they were losing some weight too. I went back to school to develop the techniques that I needed to help me take all of my experiences and become a better coach for my clients. Fresh Start Nutrition and Coaching, LLC was born!

The most difficult part of changing the way we eat initially is making the commitment as a family, but it has been my experience that we really are all in this together. That is why perfecting a few easy recipes can go a very long way in the beginning, when it comes to keeping everyone happy. When you feel better and you know it's because of the food you are eating, you want to give your family the same gift. Children are only used to what we have been giving them their whole lives and they will get used to new things as well. They also get used to feeling better and not having the sugar highs and lows. Their eating will become more consistent and they will be satisfied for longer periods of time.

When we make being healthy a family value, mindful eating becomes a cherished practice. We learn to appreciate where our food comes from and how it came to be on our plate. When we feel good it is so easy to see our blessings. When we take the time to stop the old ways we were doing and eating, and teach ourselves to taste real food again, magical things start to happen.

Moms want a lot of things and most of them have to do with our children's health and happiness. I have made it my life's mission to help as many mothers as I can see the importance of a diet rich in whole foods. The following recipes are two of my children's favorites and they often times think the sweet potato salad is dessert. The chicken veggie meatballs are a great finger food and the tomato dipping sauce is a terrific substitute for ketchup (which is full of high fructose corn syrup).

Small steps lead to big changes, and a lifetime of health is a gift we would all feel great about giving our kids!

CHICKEN VEGGIE MEATBALLS WITH ROASTED TOMATO DIPPING SAUCE

Ingredients:

FOR MEATBALLS:

- 1 lb. ground organic chicken
- 1 small organic zucchini
- 2 organic carrots
- 1/2 bunch fresh organic parsley
- Salt and pepper to taste
- Extra virgin olive oil
- 1 tbsp. lard

FOR SAUCE:

- 1 pint of assorted grape tomatoes
- 2 tbsp. fresh basil
- Maldon sea salt flakes
- Fresh ground pepper
- Extra virgin olive oil

Directions:

Preheat oven to 350.

FOR DIPPING SAUCE:

Place tomatoes in a glass pie dish and add basil. Coat tomatoes with the extra virgin olive oil and sprinkle with salt and pepper.

Bake for about an hour, tossing occasionally, and remove from the oven when the skins on the tomatoes split.

Get the tomatoes into the oven before you start the meatballs.

FOR MEATBALLS:

Peel zucchini and carrots and shred with a box cheese grater.

Cut parsley leaves into strips.

In a large bowl, combine ground chicken, zucchini, carrots, and parsley. Add salt and pepper and form mixture into meatballs.

Line a cookie sheet with parchment paper and place the meatballs on top. I like to brush meatballs with the lard or olive oil, but it isn't necessary.

Bake in the same oven as the tomatoes for 40 minutes, tossing and basting after 20 minutes. Centers should be white.

Serve meatballs on a leaf of green butter lettuce with the tomatoes on the side in a ramekin.

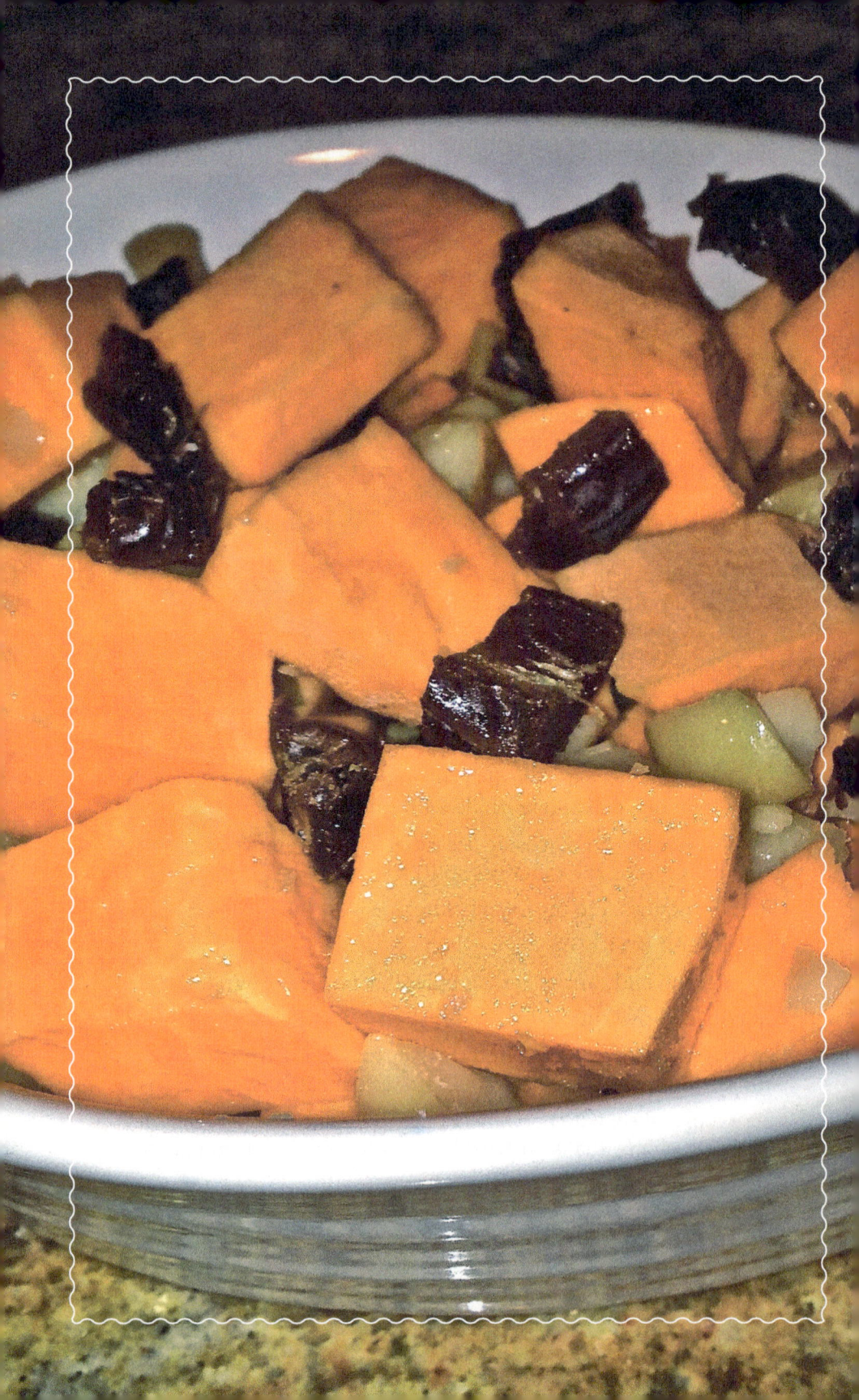

SWEET AND CRUNCHY SWEET POTATO SALAD

Ingredients:

- 4 large organic sweet potatoes
- 3 oz. organic macadamia nuts
- 4 or 5 organic Medjool dates
- Maldon sea salt flakes
- Macadamia nut oil to coat

Directions:

Peel and cube the sweet potatoes and place into an oven safe casserole dish.

Half or quarter the macadamia nuts, whatever your preference and add to the bowl with the sweet potatoes.

Drizzle the macadamia nut oil over the potatoes and nuts and toss to coat.

Sprinkle with salt flakes and bake for roughly one hour, or until brown, tossing and checking on them every 15 minutes.

While the sweet potatoes are cooking, remove the pits from the dates and slice them into eighths.

When the sweet potatoes are removed from the oven, toss the sliced dates in.

Salad may be served warm or cold.

Sherry Rothwell, RHN

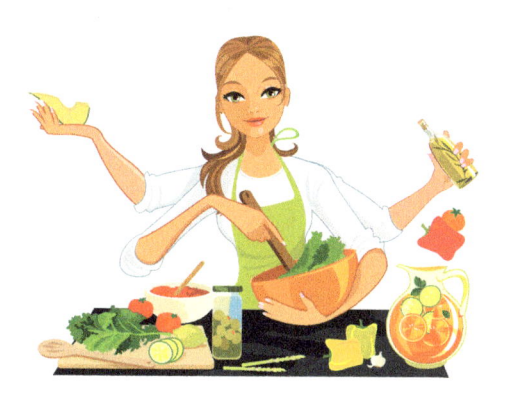

Sherry Rothwell, RHN, coaches, trains, and certifies holistic practitioners in "nutritional wisdom for the childbearing years." She provides her students and apprentices with business training and DFY (done for you) design, marketing systems, and copy templates, so that they can spend more time nurturing their families (and the women they serve) and less time in front of the computer "trying to find the right words" or figure out the whole business and marketing thing. You can learn more about working with Sherry at:

- www.NourishMama.com
- www.facebook.com/NourishMama

PRACTICE 30

Say YES! to Sweets

By Sherry Rothwell, RHN

In my early twenties, a bout with mononucleosis caused my body to really "not like" white sugar, and I would feel shooting aches and pains all over my body when I consumed anything that contained it. And worse, even a simple second cookie would crash my immune system to the point that a cold or flu would often follow.

And so I simply swore off all sugar.

Fast forward six years later and becoming a mom, the aversion to sugar stuck. When my children were small, I wouldn't even include a smoothie on the menu. I feared that even a mere tbsp. of honey would turn them into little sugar addicts!

I was always saying "no."

But then I started to notice that my food "policing" in front of friends and family, caused my kids to feel embarrassed, ashamed, and deprived. It felt bad for me too, but I didn't know what else to do. I was only trying to protect them.

After a certain age though, it becomes nearly impossible to shelter our kids from junk food.

Unless of course you want to handcuff grandma and grandpa, homeschool, or never let your kids leave the house.

I've had to let go of the reigns and reconsider what I feel to be the best approach to raising healthy kids, in spite of a society that creates obstacles to that (at seemingly every turn).

And while I would love for my children to be exposed to nothing but the wholesome traditional food of our ancestors, sadly that is just not realistic idea in today's world of fast food.

After saying no to sweets for far too, and calling certain foods bad for you or toxic, I created a lot of tension around food with my kids.

The more control I imposed, the more they pushed back. And that's when I started to hear "ew, yuck" at the dinner table a lot more than I'd care to admit. It's also when I started finding hidden junk food in my twelve-year-old son's room.

Word to the wise mama: When you say no to something or "call down" something your child wants to have or experience for themselves, they internalize that as shame (while at the same time becoming more attracted to it than ever)!

Once they are old enough, they will actually organize their lives around trying to get it. They'll either hide it from you, or even eat it just to spite you.

By focusing on what I didn't want my kids to eat, I created the very thing that my ego feared the most (especially being a nutritionist) — losing control of my children's eating habits.

If you can relate, don't worry, this doesn't have to happen in your family. You can still be a health conscious mama without creating counter-will in your kids!

It is my hope that sharing my experience with you will save you from having to learn the hard way, like I did.

If I could do it all over again, here is how I would do it:

I would let go of trying to control what other people feed my kids and simply allow them to be nourished by the social elements of enjoying food in the company of the people they love.

I would have released my worries (had I known how). Underneath the guise of perfect eating is the fear of disease. If we are confident that our children are eating healthy most of the time, why do we give so much weight and power to one plate of food that doesn't meet our standards?

I have also found within myself that the less I felt connected at the soul level with my kids, the more I fret about what they are eating... when what they really need is attention and focus on nurturing at the soul level.

Follow the 80/20 rule. Let them eat freely to their heart's desires outside of the home, yet stock your fridge with healthy and whole foods (plus an array of organic grab-and-go snacks). That way your family will eat healthy 80 percent of the time (without you having to spend a lot of time thinking about it).

I would have exercised more self-control with my words, because words are medicine. No more negative food talk. I suggest taking the words *bad*, *processed*, *toxic*, and *unhealthy* out of your day-to-day vocabulary when talking about food with your kids. Telling our kids that certain foods are toxic or bad when they are just going to eat them anyway is like forcing them to chew and swallow the fear of disease. Just zip it!

Say yes more often to treats! Make them cookies, cake, muffins, and whatever they want, just use the most nutritionally-dense ingredients: ones like butter, coconut oil, gelatin, whipped cream, cream cheese, and unrefined sugars like Rhapadura, Sucanat, and Panella instead of white sugar. Don't worry about the quantity as much as the quality. If your children are getting enough protein and fat in their diet, they will not overeat sweets. Pleasure deprivation and nutrient deficiency are the real root causes of overeating sugar.

Finally, focus on what they WILL eat, not on what they don't (or won`t). What you focus on expands, so trust your kids. See them as capable of listening to their own body. Don't hover, hold your breath, or project fear into their experience of nourishment.

If you've deprived your kids of sweets for a long time, they will likely enjoy a period of bingeing, but after the novelty wears off, they will settle back into moderation. So work on yourself, mama. Love and trust your kids. Don't teach them to fear food. Focusing on what is wrong won't make things right. So look for ways to put pleasure back on your table by saying YES! to sweets and treat those sweet little souls.

SUNSHINE YOGURT

This recipe is the perfect nutrient-dense and probiotic-promoting kid-friendly bedtime snack!

With the addition of raw egg yolks, it includes a range of nutrients so extensive, that it offers much better insurance than a daily multivitamin (most of the nutrition in an egg is found in the yolk).

This is especially so, because unlike a multivitamin, egg yolks contain DHA, which is necessary for proper brain and eye development, as well as the Omega 6 fatty acid arachidonic acid, which is required for healthy skin, hair, libido, reproduction, growth, and repair. These fatty acids are of special importance for young children and pregnant and lactating women.

Make sure to purchase pastured eggs (ones from chickens that are free to forage for grass and insects), not only to be sure that they are safe to consume raw, but of course because they are more nutritious and it makes for a more compassionate choice than purchasing eggs from chickens raised in confinement.

Ingredients:

- 1 cup yogurt
- 2 raw egg yolks (you can use save the whites to make coconut macaroons)
- honey, maple syrup, or English toffee stevia (to taste)

Directions:

Put the yogurt in a bowl.

Crack the eggs, separating out the whites.

Stir in the egg yolks and the sweetener.

Enjoy!

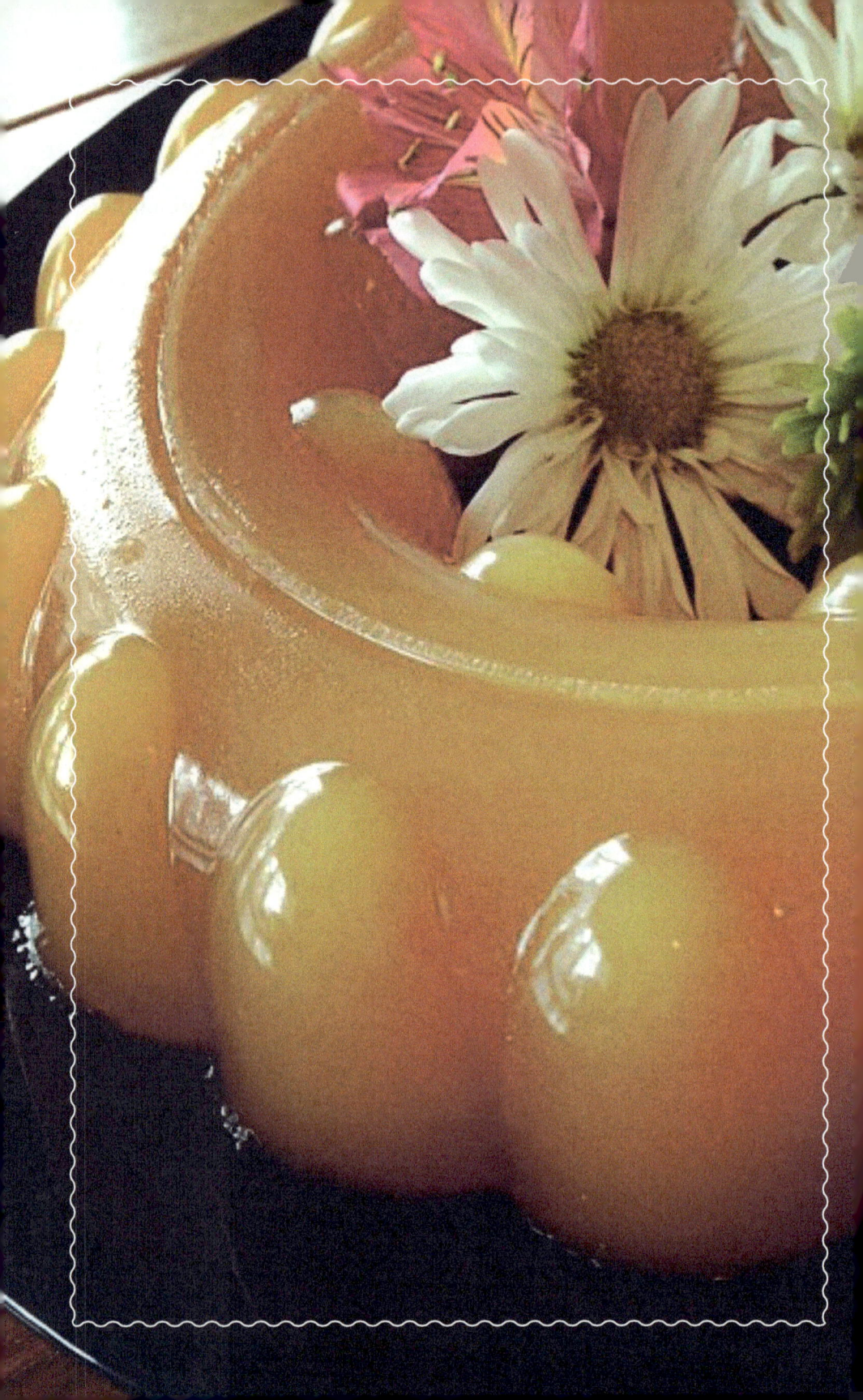

JUICE JELL-O

Want to discover the perfect alternative to conventional Jell-O and forego the sugar, food dye, and artificial flavor?

If you said yes, then you'll love this simple homemade juice Jell-O recipe.

Grass-fed gelatin (from animals raised on pasture) is not only a protein rich, nourishing, and easy-to-digest food, but it also helps to mitigate the impact of the concentrated sugars in juice by slowing down their absorption, thus preventing your child from suffering the emotional roller coaster ride of sugar highs and lows.

Gelatin is also high in glycine, an important nutrient for growth—making gelatin a must-have food for children who are slow to grow.

Ingredients:

- 1 to 2 tbsp. grass-fed gelatin (depending on how thick you want it)
- 2 cups juice

Directions:

Mix the gelatin into 1/2 cup of the fruit juice in a medium-sized saucepan on low heat.

Stir or whisk until dissolved completely.

Mix with remaining juice and pour into dish or gelatin mould

Cover with lid (or plastic wrap) and refrigerate overnight or until set.

Serve with a generous dollop of whipping cream or slightly sweetened Crème Fraiche on top for added nutrition and that grounding quality that will keep the kids calm.

Enjoy!

Conclusion

I hope you have enjoyed reading the chapters and learning about each co-author as they shared their story with you with encouragement to help moms become change agents for life. If you are like me, a visual learner, you probably really enjoyed seeing the main dish, for a better sense of the end result. We hope you enjoy this food journey.

Enjoy the process of becoming more mindful of yourself in your life, and creating a unique practice of eating with your family—honoring the body, mind and spirit. Remember to breathe through those busy moments of overthinking and recognize the importance of returning to your breath. Don't forget to laugh your way through mistakes and build on one idea of healthy cooking to the next—you're building confidence.

Take your own story of transformation and write it down. Find your favorite recipes and make them your own as you learn the skills of healthy cooking. Reach out for support and create a circle of trust where you can learn, grow, and blossom into the super mom you dream of being. Keep in mind we all start somewhere and each one of us has a unique story, journey to healing, and gifts to offer.

I want to encourage you to keep reading through this book as a reference for transformation and healthy eating. You might relate to one specific co-author and feel the urge to reach out for support. We encourage you to follow your first impression and intuition. Sometimes one particular message can change your life. Make sure to follow your body cues and listen closely to what it needs: water, rest, certain foods, love, exercise, self-care, or cleansing.

We want you to get excited about incorporating these dishes into your weekly meal plan. You can start by creating one dish a week. Experiment with your family, and let the taste testing begin! Please comment about the dishes on our website. We want to hear from you. www.balanceforbusymomscookbook.com.

COMPILED BY **HEATHER EDEN**

Join Our Tribe

Are you committed heart and soul to making necessary, permanent changes to your health and your family's health? Do you need support and a vehicle for change and awareness? Do you need coaching and support for diet and lifestyle changes, parenting, love, relationships, spirituality, intimacy, and career? Would you like to join a tribe of other likeminded moms working through a process of healing, complete wellness, and life fulfillment? Let us help you become fully awake in life. Move through mindset limitations and find your bold inner strength to persevere through life challenges and relationships. Become the best mom ever with support from like-minded moms and professionals who can bring you through an incredible transformation—mind, body, and soul. Continue this journey with us and join our "Balance for Busy Moms Tribe" for lifelong positive changes. Make your life the best you've ever dreamed of with your spouse and children. The heart matters. You matter. Learn to build a force field of love around you and your children. Learn to raise your vibration and create the most positive outcome of any circumstance. Gain the knowledge and learn the proper tools for creating the changes necessary to prevent illness, overcome stress, and adversity. Learn to properly guide your children with love, improve your home, and heal your relationships with self-compassion and service. Unite with community, learn about branding, and following your dreams for a fulfilling career and service to our planet.

Join our "Balance for Busy Moms Tribe" for unlimited access to ongoing health and wellness classes taught by experienced professionals—our co-authors—who have the secrets, keys, and strategies for success. Develop lasting friendships with other moms and take a retreat with us! Start threads on important mom matters, download workouts, eBooks, recipes, cleanses, and monthly freebies. Learn to be a kitchen goddess, find your bliss, and make your mark. Join us for a year and find out how amazing your life will transform. All classes are group coaching for an affordable price you won't find anywhere, and they are exclusively tailored for moms! Our coaches are unbelievably knowledgeable and sincere. Let's us help you reach your goals through community.

Visit www.balanceforbusymomstribe.com and join the BBM Tribe today!

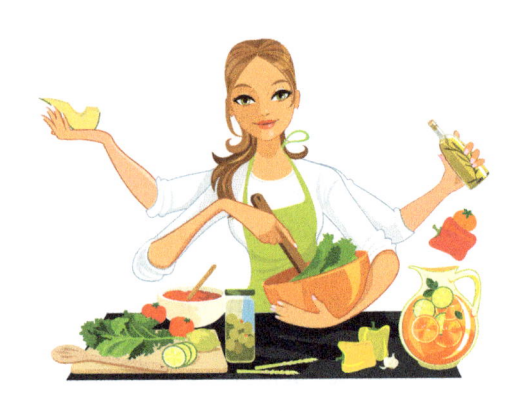

The End